60 tips

healthy skin

Catherine Maillard

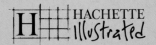

HACHETTE
Illustrated

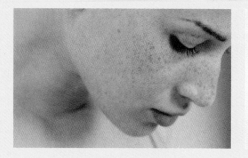

1 >>> 20
TIPS

contents

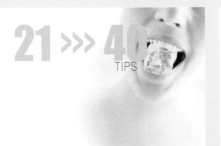

21 >>> 40
TIPS

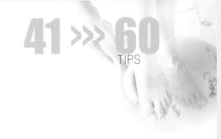

41 >>> 60
TIPS

intro
peachy skin or parchment skin?

Nowadays most of us agree that real beauty goes beyond mere appearances. But the fact remains, the first thing we tend to notice about someone is their skin. If you think of skin as not much more than the body's wrapping paper, then it's probably time you got to know it better. This book tells you, in a simple manner, everything you need to know to understand and make the most of your skin.

The skin's functions

The skin is exposed daily to numerous environmental hazards — wind, rain, extremes of temperature, pollutants — against which it provides a barrier to protect us. It also carries out certain biological functions, such as regulating the body's temperature and hydration rate. And, yes, it breathes. Its role, in short, is to receive and transmit vital information to the whole body as a means of maintaining the biological equlibrium. It has so many amazing qualities that it truly deserves all the time and care we can lavish upon it.

The three layers of the skin

The skin consists of three layers known as the epidermis, the dermis and the hypodermis, each of which has its own role and structure. Together they enable the skin to function efficiently. The epidermis, or surface layer, has two main functions: to protect the body and to expel sweat. It is composed of highly resistant cells held together by a proteinic substance called keratin. These cells constantly renew themselves, leaving the so-called 'dead cells' on the surface of the skin. The dermis, or middle layer, is the one through which we feel sensations due to the presence of papillae attached to the nerve endings. It contains collagen and elastin which create the skin's elasticity, the sweat-glands and the sebaceous (oil) glands. It is when the dermis changes that the signs of ageing appear. The hypodermis is the deepest layer of the skin and is made up of a fatty tissue that provides nourishment to the upper layers. It contains the blood vessels and nerves, conserves body heat and protects the bones and muscles, not to mention that it is the hypodermis that gives the face the firmness of its contours.

Your skin is emotive

However, the skin is not just a barrier between the body and the outside world. It is also highly sensitive to emotions. When we experience a feeling of intense happiness or a pang of unrequited love for example, the veins dilate, blood flows and the skin reddens. On the other hand, feelings of fear or jealousy will cause the veins to shrink, the blood to become sluggish and the skin to blanch and get colder. The skin is a mirror of our emotions. If it speaks, it can also scream. A grand stage for psychosomatic illnesses, it also has a special talent for dramatizing the subconscious. Acne, hives, psoriasis: these are just a few of its expresssions. So we can conclude that skincare is much more than simply taking care of the appearance.

Recent studies have confirmed the link between the skin and the psyche. We know that the nervous system and the skin share a common tissue, coming as they both do from the ectoderm which is the outermost of the three primal layers of an embryo. Skin and nervous system only begin to separate three weeks after conception. Hardly surprising then that we have a strong sense of the connection between the skin and the feelings, and even more reason to be kind to our skin.

Take care of yourself

Rich in sense-receptors, the skin can detect and react with outside influences, so good skincare is not just maintaining the beauty of the epidermis but also involves your overall health. A beautiful skin has a silky feel, clear contours and a sprinkle of glamour; but even the best products can only be fully effective if you keep to a good cleansing regime and healthy eating habits. The secret of a good skin lies in knowing how to make use of your natural allies. Whether your skin is dry, oily or tired, you need to understand its needs and adapt your regime to suit it. A consultation with an aesthetician or a dermatologist can establish a precise diagnosis of your skin profile and is a good start on the way to achieving your full potential.

Make the right choices

You can buy up the entire cosmetic department of your favourite shop to make yourself feel luxurious but only if you know how to adapt to the season. Your skin's needs are different in winter, spring and summer; so too should be the products and the methods you choose. If nothing seems to work for a certain problem (deep lines or psoriasis for example) refer to the chapters on different weather conditions and you can adjust your regime accordingly. Whatever your dermatological profile, you will find hundreds of ideas here which will help you realize your dream complexion: don't use them sparingly!

how to use this book

This book offers a made-to-measure programme, which will enable you to deal with your own particular problem. It is organized into four sections:

• **A questionnaire** to help you to assess the extent of your problem.
• **The first 20 tips** that will show you how to change your daily life in order to prevent problems and maintain health and fitness.
• **20 slightly more radical tips** that will develop the subject and enable you to cope when problems occur.
• **The final 20 tips** which are intended for more serious cases, when preventative measures and attempted solutions have not worked.

At the end of each section someone with the same problem as you shares his or her experiences.

You can go methodically through the book from tip 1 to 60 putting each piece of advice into practice. Alternatively, you can pick out the recommendations which appear to be best suited to your particular case, or those which fit most easily into your daily routine. Or, finally, you can choose to follow the instructions according to whether you wish to prevent stress problems occuring or cure ones that already exist.

what skin type are you?

Answer the following questions honestly by ticking the   or   box, according to whether you are rarely or regularly affected by these problems.

YOUR SKIN'S APPEARANCE

yes	no	1	Is your skin permanently dull-looking?
yes	no	2	Do you make sure that cleanse your skin every morning?
yes	no	3	Do you suffer from dryness and red patches at the first sign of winter?
yes	no	4	Do you have dry cheeks and a shiny nose?

YOUR BEHAVIOUR PATTERN

yes	no	5	Are you a real sun worshipper?
yes	no	6	Does what you eat tend to reflect the needs of your skin?
yes	no	7	Do you take any exercise?
yes	no	8	Do you respect the natural biological rhythms of your skin?

YOUR DAILY CARE REGIME

yes	no	9	Are you familiar with the uses of essential oils for the skin?
yes	no	10	Have you thought about anti-wrinkle treatments?
yes	no	11	Do you take a copper supplement when you have skin problems?
yes	no	12	Are you into treatments based on exotic plants?

If you replied **yes**
to questions 2, 7, 8 and 9,
refer to Tips **1** to **20**.
If you replied **yes**
to questions 1, 4, 5 and 10,
look at Tips **21** to **40**.
If you replied **yes**
to questions 3, 6, 11 and 12
refer to Tips **41** to **60**.

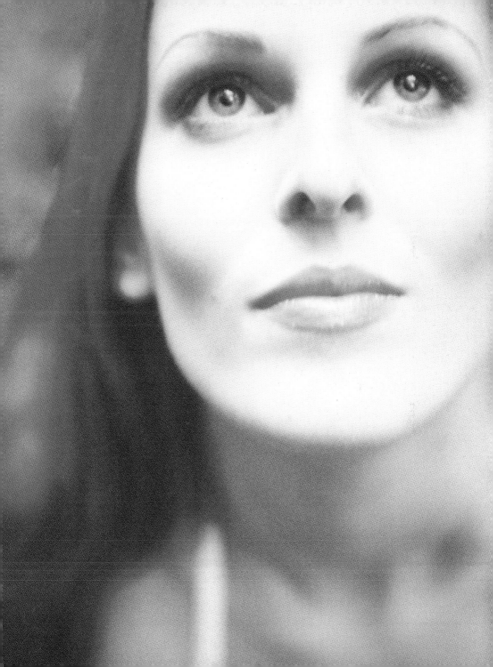

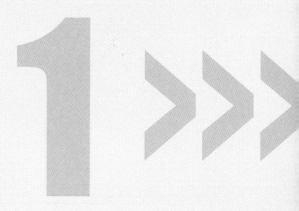

>> **You have healthy skin and you want to keep it that way.** Good, then you need only read the following tips and apply them on a daily basis. If you maintain a regular beauty regime, you can easily improve both the tone and firmness of your skin.

>>>> **After a long, difficult day, all you want to do is slip into a smooth, freshly-ironed skin and rest your beautiful face on the pillow.** It sounds idyllic and is not impossible. By following the simplest of routines on a daily basis, you can achieve this.

>>>>>> **Our beauty regime depends on natural treatments** and the gentlest of care. Your skin will become much more luminous.

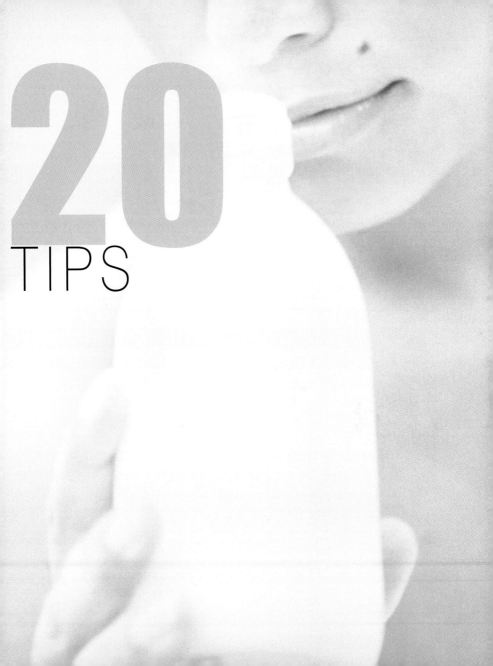

20

TIPS

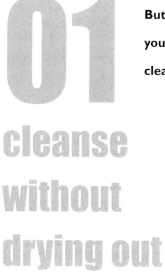

01
cleanse
without
drying out

Removal of every last trace of make-up is the first step on the road to a beautiful complexion. But, be sure that you use products which suit your own skin type and needs. This is the key to cleansing properly.

Morning routine

When you get up in the morning cleanse your skin – this should always be the first part of your beauty regime. Took your make-up off the night before? So, do it again! Cleansers get rid of dirt and grease as well as make-up itself. Choose the type which best suits your skin.

● ● ● DID YOU KNOW?

> Warm an amount of your creamy cleanser in the palm of your hand before applying on your face. Then gently massage it into your skin using a circular motion. Press with the palms to remove the impurities and wipe off with paper tissue.

> If you use a toner, remove all traces of it with a cotton wool, wiping your skin repeatedly.
> If you have very dry skin, don't cleanse in the morning so you retain the oils secreted during the night.

Creams

The new cream-based cleansers are ideal for dry or sensitive skins and leave them feeling fresh. Their hydrating, nourishing properties leave a protective layer on the surface of your skin. Follow with a toning lotion for best results.

Foaming cleansers

If you prefer to wash your face with water, then foaming cleansers are a good option. They cleanse without using soap, and must be rinsed off with plenty of water. They contain gentle surface-active agents which do not strip the skin of its natural oils and have calcium sensors to prevent tautness. Foaming cleansers are good for dry and combination skin.

Cleansing milks

For those with very sensitive skin, cleansing milks are a simple and comforting option, and they do not require rinsing. They trap impurities whilst leaving a soothing hydrating film on your skin.

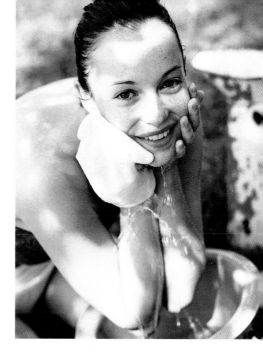

KEY FACTS

* Cleansing milks are a comforting solution for those with dry skin.

* Creams gently remove all traces of impurity from sensitive skins.

* Foaming cleansers suit those with combination skin and leave the skin really clean.

02

Your eyes are one of the most delicate organs in the body. When cleansing be sure to choose products carefully and treat your eyes with extra gentleness.

respect your eyes

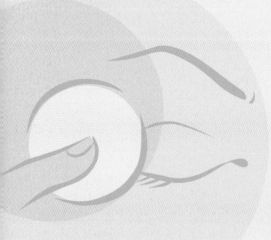

Take care of your eyes

Beauty is seen in the eyes. A few extra minutes each day will keep your eyes sparkling. Careful cleansing of the eye area should be an integral part of your daily routine and can be an agreeable and relaxing way to end the day. Remember also that the fragile tissue around the eyes can be damaged by lack of proper care. Get into the habit of always including your eyes in your beauty programme.

Choosing a make-up remover

There are various types of make-up remover to suit a wide range of lifestyles and people.

• If you're pushed for time, water-based make-up removers clean the eyes in one quick sweep of cotton wool with no need to rinse. They are also ideal for getting rid of all traces of oil.

• If you wear very little make-up, the two-phase lotions, half-cleanser half-toner, are good for you. Also suitable for sensitive skins, they leave the eyes clear and refreshed.

• If you like extra-gentle cleansing or if you don't like using water, it's best to use one of the cleansing milks. These are also recommended for the removal heavy of make-up.

●●● DID YOU KNOW?

> Cleanse eyelids and lashes with cotton wool, using a sweeping movement from the base of the nose to the temple. Remove all traces of make-up with a cotton bud soaked in cleanser. Rinse with a gentle toner.

> Professional make-up artists advise against removing make-up if you need to reapply it straight away, as there tends to be a transfer of the old make-up into the new.

> After removing your make-up, take a few minutes to massage your eyes. Close your eyes and cover with both hands, pressing lightly against the eyeballs with the palms. Take a few deep breaths, relax.

KEY FACTS

* Choose your make-up remover according to your personal needs.

* Learn to pamper your eyes.

* Use cotton buds for delicate areas.

* Never reapply make-up immediately after removal.

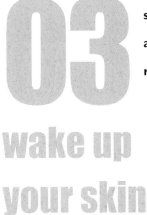

03

wake up your skin

Water is vital to awaken your skin – not only the water you drink but also the water you splash on your face. A healthy breakfast and a gentle massage will help your skin have a rosy glow at the start of the day.

The first drops of water

Do you consider that your skin's beauty starts from the moment you open your eyes in the morning? If not, then you need convincing that this is the case. You can start the hydration process of your cells even before you get up, by drinking a few sips of fresh mineral water. Water is indispensable for the elimination of toxins and revitalization of your body. Once you get up, splash your face first with tepid and then cold water, cupping it in your hands. Thirty seconds should be enough to remove any signs of sleep from your face. If you have a fragile, sensitive skin, a mineral-water spray is a good option.

Air and massage

In order to oxygenate your skin and to trigger circulation, try the following breathing exercise. Breathe in whilst inflating your stomach and then slowly exhale, pushing out all the oxygen from your lungs.

A quick facial massage will allow you to face the day with relaxed features:

• Use the tips of your fingers to gently massage a little day cream around your eyes and mouth.

• Gently pinch your cheeks with your fingertips to produce a rosy glow. Then moisturize your skin.

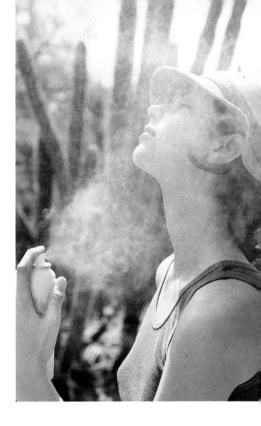

> Cereals rich in fatty acids protect and nourish the skin. Wheat makes it smoother and oats reinforce the intercellular cement, thereby preventing excessive loss of water.

KEY FACTS

* Drink plenty of water to maintain a healthy glow.

* Breathe deeply to oxygenate your skin.

* Prepare a breakfast for your skin.

04 hydrate your skin thoroughly

Even if you have a good complexion, it won't stay that way forever if it isn't properly hydrated. Always choose a day cream to suit your skin type.

> Try anti-wrinkle patches. These can revitalize the skin by draining and hydrating the areas where fine lines appear and protect it against drying out.

●●● DID YOU KNOW?

> Always choose a cream specially formulated for your skin type. Apply morning and night and try not to skip this part of your beauty regime.

Hydrated skin is younger-looking skin

Hydration is essential to hold back the signs of ageing and is the key to young-looking skin. Like the body, the skin is made up of 70% water and 13% corneal layer. Below this threshold the skin weakens and is at greater risk of deterioration. Exposed to sun, wind and pollution, the corneal layer dries out and wrinkles appear. It is therefore essential to maintain the water content of the skin by thorough hydration.

To the rescue

There are several ways to replenish hydration. First and foremost, you must drink plenty of water. Remember that internal hydration takes care of 30 to 40% of the skin's needs.

To hydrate your skin from the outside, use a good cream. Applied daily, it will restore vitality.

The first casualty of dehydration is dry skin. For this, the rescue remedy is found in ceramides and fatty acids, both of which have deep penetrating properties and enrich the weakened corneal layer.

A word of warning: oily skin can also become dehydrated. In this case, you must rehydrate without adding oil. Certain products of marine origin which contain continuous skin-irrigating ingredients are best for this.

KEY FACTS

* Choose a cream which has rich hydrating properties.

* Don't forget that oily skin can be dehydrated too.

* Drink plenty of water to irrigate your skin from within.

> For lasting irrigation of the skin, nothing beats a hydrating mask. Apply to the face and neck and leave to act for at least twenty minutes. For best results, use once a week.

05

discover trace elements

We now know that what we eat has a definite effect on the skin, thanks largely to trace elements. It is therefore important to ensure you get enough trace elements in the form of food or creams.

The role of trace elements

Oligotherapy, as it is called, uses tiny amounts of mineral substances generally deriving from metals. Cosmetics experts are increasingly turning to this in the development of beauty programmes. It's a sad fact of life that we age every minute; however, by activating certain enzymes, trace elements can help to suppress the cellular oxidation which causes the skin to age. Potassium is known primarily for its diuretic action but is also vital in balancing the hydrous exchanges carried out by the skin. Selenium is good for eliminating free radicals, whilst silicon is important in maintaining the skin's elasticity. Zinc is known for its valuable healing properties and antioxidants.

How to use these treatments

Our bodies are unable to produce micronutrients. So we have to absorb them in the form of food supplements or cosmetic products. The idea of combining interior and exterior health care is almost commonplace nowadays: you need only look in your local pharmacy to see the wide range of creams, lotions, milks and gels. When using these, always ensure you follow the instructions carefully.

For additional anti-ageing care you can incorporate trace elements with the vitamins A, C, E and B6 to act as synergy. But don't forget that one of the first principles of beauty is good nourishment. Fresh fruit and vegetables, in particular, constitute excellent sources of trace elements.

● ● ● DID YOU KNOW?

> Choose trace elements according to your skin type.

• Oily skin: take zinc to regulate cellular activity and to control the secretion of sebum.

• Oily skin with a tendency to erupt: sulphur is good thanks to its ability to eliminate toxins.

• Tired or stretched-looking skin: take selenium to help combat cellular ageing.

> Be patient when using creams enriched with trace elements. You will need to apply them every day for a minimum of two months before you begin to see results.

KEY FACTS

* Following a health programme incorporating trace elements helps slow down the ageing process.

* Become more beautiful through your diet.

* For best results, combine internal and external beauty care.

06

find out the virtues of fruit

Strawberries, apples and grapes – fruit-based cosmetics are all the rage. Face masks or creams using fruit acids are part of nature's treasure. Your skin will love you if you use them.

Multi-tasking molecules

AHAs (Alpha Hydroxy Acids or fruit acids) have revolutionized the cosmetic industry. Extracts of apple, sugar cane or whey are low-density moisturizers and powerful exfoliators. They play a two-pronged role, hydrating the dry outer layer of skin whilst cleansing it and stimulating cell renewal. They are highly effective in removing the dead layer

● ● ● D I D   Y O U   K N O W ?

> Oily skins like fruit acids, whereas dry skins can pull and redden with their use. Use a product with only 8% fruit acid content for a few weeks to start with. If your skin reddens, apply less frequently.

> OPCs (oligomeric proanthocyanidins) are also part of nature's harvest. Grape-seed extracts are excellent protectors of collagen and

of skin and introducing a healthy new glow to your face. Studies have shown that AHAs promote the production of collagen and can help your skin to retain its elasticity.

Using AHAs properly

Fruit acids can be found in many moisturizers. Enjoy a course of treatment lasting three months and wait a few weeks before embarking on another one. AHAs are also available in masks and give your skin an instant boost.
Before you go out in the sun, apply a total sunscreen to your face if using fruit acid products. They can make your skin more sensitive to the sun by thinning the top layer of skin.

elastin. Their antioxidant properties are 200 times greater than those of Vitamin E.

KEY FACTS

* To regain your skin's elasticity, try using fruit acids.

* Alternate between AHA creams and masks and your normal moisturizer.

* Try products which contain grape-seed extracts for their anti-ageing properties.

07

explore
the power
of water

Although not quite the same as using freshly-collected rainwater, water therapy is nonetheless effective in replenishing thirsty skin. Clever use of mineral water will give your skin a real home cure.

Thermal springs in a bottle

Hard, calcareous water is bad for the skin. If you have sensitive or easily irritated skin you should resort to nature for your daily skin care. Ranges of thermal and mineral waters contain trace elements, although each water has different properties.

Natural benefits are intensified, sometimes by as much as ten times, by the cosmetic additives in thermal water.

● ● ● DID YOU KNOW?

> Using a mineral-water atomizer is still the best way to achieve freshness. Simply substitute for your usual toner. It can also be used after applying make-up to fix and prolong its wear. Or, spray on any time of the day when you need to add a little freshness to your skin.

> Hold the spray about 20cm (8in) away from your face, spray, then leave to act for two to three minutes before drying. This is an ideal way to maintain the hydration of your skin.

Once you accept that hydration is one of the skin's most basic needs, it should no longer seem an extravagance to give yourself a home spa.

Good use of water therapy

The best way to retain water in the cutaneous tissues remains the application of a water- therapy treatment directly onto the skin. There are numerous formulas available and they have been produced with the express purpose of aiding the cell renewal of body and skin. Apply as you would an ordinary spray atomizer to cleanse or simply refresh the face; then leave to dry naturally in the air; finally blotting with a paper tissue. This will leave a protective film on the skin and a feeling of total comfort. Used in the evening as a relaxant or in the morning as a toner, water therapy is a friend to your skin.

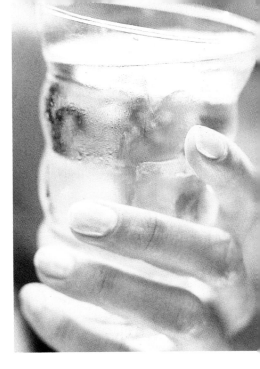

> If you suffer from rosacea, apply a soothing thermal or mineral water compress directly onto your face.

KEY FACTS

* Thermal water treatments enliven the complexion.

* Water therapy also contains hydrating agents that help to counteract dryness.

* The composition of thermal waters is very close to the skin's own.

08 try thalasso-therapy

Beauty may be skin deep but it also comes from the deep – the sea. Let's look at the properties found in seaweed, which literally swims in marine goodness.

> Famous for its relaxant properties, brown shore seaweed (Ascophyllum nodosum) is an excellent as a cure for stress.
> Californian blue seaweed (Spirula maxima) combats fatigue and slows down cellular ageing.

The virtues of seaweed

Seaweed plays an important role in natural beauty care. This versatile marine plant contains a high concentration of salts, minerals, vitamins and trace elements. Our own fluid organs (blood, lymph, plasma) contain properties very similar to those found in seaweed. Among the most interesting seaweeds are Ulva undaria and Porphyra, full of exceptional powers to combat free radicals and helpful in promoting a velvet skin; then there is Sanguinea delestria, rich in vitamins A and K, and particularly effective in hydration. The regular use of seaweeds in the form of creams or masks provides a preventative and curative action against ageing for the skin.

Thalassotherapy and its role in your regime

For protecting the skin against the hazards of modern living (stress, pollution etc.) nothing beats a truly iodized rest. If you want to rediscover your beauty, lissomness and 'joie de vivre' then give yourself a thalassotherapy break. It is a completely natural cure which combines many benefits of the sea and rejuvenates both mind and body. The star of the show is seawater, rich in trace elements (chlorine, sodium, magnesium, calcium etc.), which, in a bath, penetrates into the body through the skin. For best results, the seawater should be heated to a temperature of 32 to 33°C (60 to 62°F). If at all possible, take two or three short cures every year – this will have the same effect as a mini facelift.

> To choose the best treatment for you, read the labels carefully or consult your pharmacist.
> A thalasso bath will invigorate the whole body. Soak for fifteen to twenty minutes and wrap up in a warm bathrobe afterwards.

KEY FACTS

* Choose cosmetic products containing seaweed.

* Thalasso cures work like a mini facelift.

* Plunge into a seaweed bath to re-mineralize your skin.

09 grow beautiful whilst you dream

At night, whilst we sleep, the cells divide twice as quickly and it is then that the skin performs most of its recovery. Regular use of a night cream maximizes the benefits.

During the night Your skin is subject to a lot of wear during the day, so it is essential you take good care of it at night to help the process of cell regeneration. This is when the cells at the deeper layers come through and transform into surface cells, rich in keratin.

Night creams Opt for a night cream that is more nourishing and hydrating than your day cream. The day cream works as a defence against the environment and the night cream acts as a regenerator. Go for the formulas rich in essential fatty acids that nourish the hydro-lypidic film. Creams containing vitamins A, C and E combat free radicals. For the best results, it is important to respect the biological rhythm of your skin: the best time for applying night-time skincare is before midnight.

● ● ● DID YOU KNOW?

> Lack of sleep is immediately visible in the skin in the form of dullness, lines and dark rings.
> Never skimp on your night-time ritual of cleansing, toning and nourishing and night cream. Drink a long glass of water before you go to sleep and another one immediately on waking.

KEY FACTS

✳ At night help your skin to recharge its batteries by using a night cream or balm.

✳ Get enough sleep. Your skin needs it.

10 lift with serums

We all have bad skin days when no matter what we do, the face looks old and tired. Now, thanks to the latest advances in skincare, help is at hand. Serums are here to lift the skin and bring about active regeneration.

Toning is essential. All skin types need toning to help them resist loss of firmness. With time, the contours of the face naturally begin to sag and lose their definition. The process of regeneration begins to slow and the muscles of the face retract.

Choose products that lift the skin. It is better not to wait for the signs of ageing to appear before thinking about taking action. Serums consist of highly concentrated biological ingredients designed to drain, tighten and lift the skin almost instantaneously.

● ● ● DID YOU KNOW?

> Keep your serum in the refrigerator. It will be even more effective in stabilizing and firming the skin.
> Reinforce the action of the serum by including the use of fresh water in your beauty ritual.

KEY FACTS

* Tiredness and the effects of the weather visibly drag down the skin.

* Don't wait too long before trying a serum.

* Serums work so effectively and quickly thanks to their extremely concentrated active ingredients.

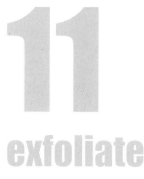

11
exfoliate

Sun damage, pollution, tiredness ... your skin ends up exhausted. In addition to your daily beauty routine you should sometimes give your skin an intensive purifying treatment. The way to do this is to exfoliate.

Purify by scrubbing

Exfoliation is actually a natural process by which the skin rids itself of its dead cells. But sometimes we need to help nature along a little for the following reasons: when you are young the average cycle of skin rejuvenation is between 20 and 28 days, however this process becomes increasingly slow with age. Add to that the various environmental nasties we face daily (sun, pollution etc.) that make the cells multiply in excess, gradually suffocating the skin and giving it a dull appearance. Regular use of an exfoliant allows you to remove these impurities and give back the skin its luminosity.

Exfoliators

Exfoliators are most commonly composed of tiny granules which, when massaged on the skin, get rid of blackheads and dead cells. The massage effect stimulates the circulation so aiding the intercellular renewal process, and the skin appears radiant again.
There is another type of exfoliator which, instead of using granules, works by transforming itself on application into a soft paste giving an effective but gentler treatment.
The AHA (fruit acid) creams also work well as exfoliants, leaving the complexion smooth and clear.

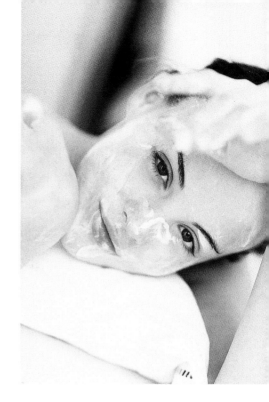

> Then immerse your body in the water, rinse and reapply the oil.

KEY FACTS

* Regular use of an exfoliator is essential.

* Exfoliants come in granular or paste form, or as fruit acids.

* Use of exfoliators (regularity, pressure of application) should be judged according to skin type.

12

uncover the magic of masks

Hydrating beauty masks are amazing. Because they are highly concentrated and super-absorbent you need only use a tiny amount from time to time to get good results. The secret behind their efficacy lies in the active ingredients which adjust themselves to the needs of the epidermis.

Why should I use a mask?

Masks can dramatically improve the features no matter how old you are or what type of skin you have. In responding to the needs of the epidermis, they reverse the harmful effects of weather conditions whilst toning and hydrating the skin. For optimum results alternate products which contain different ingredients. Use a clay mask to purify; a thermal mask to sooth the skin; vitamin C to revitalise; apricot oil to hydrate...

Masking your face in beauty

You should use a mask once a week or more frequently if you love their refreshing and regenerative effect. Always try to avoid the delicate area around the eyes when applying. Instead apply liberally to the neck- a highly delicate part of the body often overlooked in everyday beauty care. Take care to stick to the time indicated on the product as taking it off too quickly will not give it time to work properly and leaving it on too long can produce the exact opposite of the desired effect – which is, to enable the skin to adapt to its environment by balancing itself naturally.

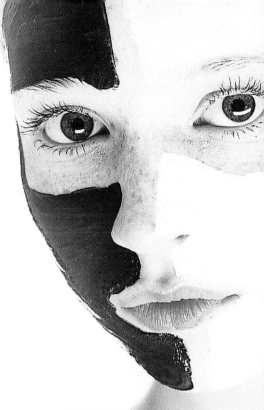

> Make the most of your beauty session by listening to some peaceful background music. Choose sounds from nature: birds, animals, the sea. Think multi-sensory.

 KEY FACTS

* Use a mask every time you want a beauty pick-me-up.

* Remember that a mask is twice as concentrated as a day or night cream.

* Choose your mask according to your needs: for soothing, hydrating or revitalizing.

13 find the answer in plant extracts

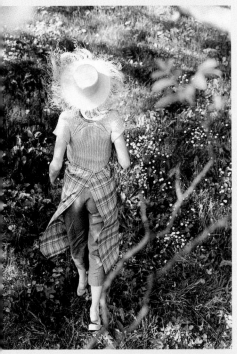

When the body is in need of equilibrium there is nothing more effective than nature. Beauty finds the answer in fields and meadows. Each essential oil possesses its own specific properties and has its own place in cosmetic use. Sage, rosemary, thyme...plants make us beautiful.

● ● ● DID YOU KNOW?

> Use sage for troubled skin. A natural antiperspirant, it possesses soothing properties effective in the treatment of redness and spots.

> For sensitive skin try neroli which brightens the complexion.
> Angelica compensates for deficiency of lipid in dry skin.
> Rosemary regulates the sebaceous secretions and tightens pores.

Essential oils

Essential oils are the extracts of aromatic plants. These perfumed liquids contain active ingredients which are concentrated up to a hundred times. Powerful and varied, they have attracted the interest of numerous cosmetic laboratories thanks to their versatility and the varying degrees of strength with which they work to oxegenate and regenerate the skin. The combination of several different essential oils reinforces the action of each one separately. You can even prepare your own beauty products according to your own particular wants. Remember that the areas in the brain which register the scents are also the ones where the centre of the emotions are found. So by using aromatic plant oils you will enhance your outer and your inner beauty simultaneously.

> Cinammon improves the skin's suppleness and elasticity.
> Use geranium as a skin pick-me-up, and rose for rebalancing.

Your beauty ritual

The key feature of the essential oils is their ability to be absorbed rapidly into the epidermis and the deeper layers of the skin. They stimulate the circulation of the blood, eliminate toxins and speed up recovery according to the active ingredients used. A word of warning: essential oils are highly concentrated and require care in their use. Start by mixing the product (7 drops) into a tablespoon of oil. Then apply delicately to the face and neck taking care to avoid the eye area.

KEY FACTS

* Essential oils respect the skin's ecosystem.

* Look to nature for all the essential oils you need to enhance your beauty.

* Create your own treatments combining different plant elements according to your needs.

14

nourish with vegetable oils

Soya, jojoba, almond ... beauty is nourished by nature. Women have been using vegetable (plant) oils since time immemorial. The unsaturated fatty acids found in these oils nourish the skin wonderfully.

Get into the vegetable oil habit

Because vegetable oils are beauty products in their pure state, they provide an intense essence of the fruit, tree or flower which they come from. Applied to the skin, they bond with the cutaneous tissue which then draws out the fatty acids essential to its nutrition. Their virtues are many: they reinforce the structure of the corneal layer and they restore the lipidic film to the epidermis. Thus protected, the skin is better hydrated and more resistant to environmental nasties.

Whether for body, hair or skin, vegetable oil is one of the most sensual treatments you can give yourself. After a bath or shower apply to a slightly damp skin as an alternative to body lotion.

Each oil has its own unique property

Soothing and softening, almond oil works wonders as a cleanser for sensitive or very dry skin.

- **Jojoba oil** regulates the secretion of sebum whilst revitalizing and nourishing the the the skin through to the dermis. In its natural form it contains a sunscreen of factor 5.
- **Evening primrose oil** and borage oil are both naturally rich in fatty acids and are equally good for skin regeneration and stabilizing the hormones.
- **Apricot kernel oil** is good for excessively oily skin.

15 detox with clay masks

Clay is a key addition to the list of beauty treatments using 100% natural ingredients. White, pink or green clay all have uses as skin detoxifiers.

In search of the natural Clay is an extremely effective natural beauty product. A sedimentary rock which derives from the slow decomposition of granite, it is made up of silicates hydrated with aluminium. Its cosmetic properties and colour are determined by the minerals (iron oxide, salts, calcium, trace elements) that have infiltrated into it.

Whatever its colour, it is rich in skin-enhancing properties and is exceptionally efficient in draining the skin of its impurities and stimulating the blood and the lymphatic system. White clay – the most neutral of the clays – is most suitable for normal or combination skin, whilst green clay is recommended for oily skin types.

Directions for use Apply a fine layer to the face and neck with the fingertips avoiding the immediate eye area. Allow to dry naturally. When you feel the mask start to pull the skin, remove with cotton wool moistened with mineral oil.

● ● ● D I D Y O U K N O W ?

> To make up a mask, pour 2 to 3 tablespoons of your chosen clay into an china or earthenware bowl (not metal). Add 3 tablespoons of mineral water. Stir until a thick paste is formed. Leave to stand for 1 hour before applying.

K E Y F A C T S

* For deep facial cleansing, use a clay mask.

* Clay draws out impurities and stimulates the circulation of the blood.

16 eat healthily

To continue your quest for beauty without wrinkles, you must ensure you are getting enough vitamins. Fresh fruit and vegetables, whole cereals – the order of the day should be quality and variety.

The importance of good nutrition B-group vitamins are indispensible in cell renewal. We know also that the best anti-wrinkle vitamins are A, C and E and beta-carotene (pro-vitamin A) which protect against the free radicals that cause ageing.

Eat wisely Green vegetables (artichokes, aubergines/egg plant, celery, broccoli, spinach) are rich in vitamin E, zinc and silicon and they rehydrate the skin from the inside. Fruit and vegetables of an orange colour contain vitamin A and beta-carotene.

Fruits which have a husk (almonds and walnuts, for example) are mines of vitamin E. Whole cereals are excellent sources of B vitamins.

KEY FACTS

* Go for the natural anti-wrinkle vitamins – A, C, E and F.

* Brighten your complexion with B group vitamins.

* Eat raw fruit and vegetables seasoned with vegetable oil.

17

get moving!

To keep yourself looking good, there's no substitute for a sporting activity. Whether alone or as a group activity, practising a sport will give you a great shape and a healthy outlook. Also, kept well oxygenated, your skin will be better than ever.

Physical activity brings contentment

Beauty is all about balance. The body, mind and skin should all be in harmony. For a good figure and healthy skin, exercise is the answer. Recent studies have shown that physical activity is an essential factor in psychological well-being. What it does, in fact, is to release endorphines which are natural mood-lifters and anti-fatigue molecules. You feel better, therefore you look better.

● ● ● DID YOU KNOW?

> Practise deep and even breathing in time with the rhythm of the exercises. Inhale before you begin and exhale during the exertion, then repeat immediately.

> Drink between 250 to 500ml (8 to 17fl oz) of water at the end of the session to dilute the lactic acid accumulated during the muscular activity.

The exertion of physical exercise also improves the circulation of the blood and maintains the musclular mass. This, in turn, activates the regeneration of the cutaneous cells and helps the face keep its shape.

Sports à la carte

Choose any sporting activity whatsoever. If you want to be more beautiful, more toned and more radiant, you should above all choose a sport which you enjoy. Don't bother with barbells in the gym if you prefer swimming in warm water! For a brighter complexion, nothing beats outdoor activities: the breathing of fresh air speeds up the oxygen supply to the skin and gets rid of dead cells. You might want to consider taking up a gentle gymnastic sport such as yoga, tai-chi or qi gong which will reduce tension and liberate your energy. These are fabulous for the complexion.

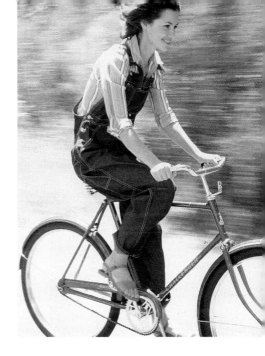

> **Never overstretch yourself: if you feel pain it's because you are pushing your body too far.**

KEY FACTS

* Sport is the key to your well-being as it improves mind, body and skin.

* A regular sporting activity produces a better oxygenization of the skin and activates the circulation of the blood.

* To look your best, always choose a sport you enjoy doing.

18

say goodbye to stress

It's difficult to escape stress in the modern world, surrounded as we all are by problems and pressures. But you can do it. Don't let stress get a grip on your skin! There are dozens of ways to keep cool, calm and collected and so preserve your inner and outer beauty.

Relaxation is an art

Do you feel tense and anxious, as if life is running you and you are not running it? To get back your sense of well-being, it's essential you learn to relax. Relaxation is an art, and its first principle is muscular control. Cramp and other disagreeable tensions often lead to more serious problems such as back trouble, indigestion and insomnia, to name but a few.

● ● ● DID YOU KNOW?

> Indulge yourself in a Zen bath filled with anti-stress essential oils, such as benzoin (from the benzoin tree cultivated in Java, Sumatra and Thailand), sandalwood, neroli or lavender.

> Unwind with a cooling eye mask whenever you feel stress overtaking you.

> Pick yourself up with a tiger-balm oil massage. This famous Chinese ointment contains a super-relaxing combination of camphor, menthol and eucalyptus.

They will be sure to keep the smile off your face and drain away your beauty.

Learn to relax

There are diverse relaxation techniques. One of the most simple is autogenic training. Lie down in a darkened room, close your eyes and breathe, inflating your stomach with air. Feel your body unwind after each movement. Tell yourself that you are feeling completely calm. Feel your body getting heavy, then hot, then colder; observe yourself with detachment, as though you are outside your body.

With a little practice, the simple fact of just saying one of these phrases to yourself will be enough to relieve your tension; and you can do this anywhere, in any situation.

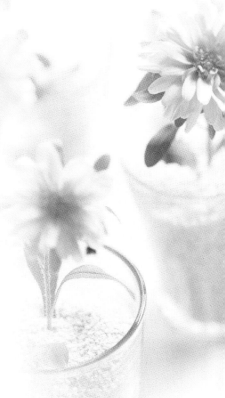

> Caress your neurones. Get a fountain for your home so you can listen to the tranquil sounds of water.

19

breathe in, breathe out

You can camouflage an unhealthy face but it's much better to oxygenate your skin properly by filling your lungs when breathing. For really healthy and restorative breathing, go walking in the countryside and sing whenever possible.

Walk in the countryside

Your skin needs to get away from city life from time to time and the perfect anti- dote to this is a walk in the countryside. Walking increases the volume of air you inhale by 20 to 30 %, which is where the feeling of revival, known to ramblers, comes from. Also the oxygen emitted by the vegetation is rich in negative ions which stimulate the dilation of the veins,

● ● ● DID YOU KNOW?

> To get the maximum benefit from breath- ing whilst singing, try to visualize the air and the sound as they are travelling along the vertebral column. This will give you a feeling of well-being which in turn will illu- minate your skin.

> For really effective abdominal breathing, try to smell the air which enters and leaves your nostrils. Then follow its progression into the inside of your olfactory organs.

increase oxygenation of the tissues and thus fights stress. It is an excellent way to wake up your appearance.

Sing for your skin

An ideal way to start the day is by singing. You will find it lifts your skin as well as your spirits. When you sing, you automatically breathe with your stomach, which is the deepest kind of breathing and the best for getting rid of tension. It also ensures better oxygenation of the skin. To hold a note, you have to breathe correctly. This is why singing revitalizes the whole of your body. It also exercises all the muscles of your face and thus helps prolong youthful features and skin elasticity.

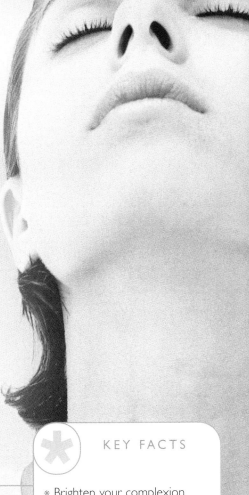

> The air you breathe in should swell up your abdomen. When you breathe out raise your diaphragm and hollow your abdomen to expel the air out of your body.

KEY FACTS

* Brighten your complexion by taking regular walks in the countryside.

* Sing to exercise all the muscles of your face.

* Oxygenate your skin through abdominal breathing.

20 practise positive thinking

Nowadays it's fashionable to look happy. Smiling has become the cosmetic norm and perfumes are specifically formulated to alter your mood. Take a few simple measures and you can feel on top of the world again.

Be cheerful Smiling is simply the best anti-wrinkle treatment of all. When you wake up tired there's no point in worrying about it, just make sure you get a good night's sleep the next night. To banish the blues on the way to the office, think of three things which will light up your day: the flowers in your garden, funny stories your colleague told you, your evening bath.

Lift your spirits with perfume There is a huge range of perfumes now available, so there is simply no need to use the same one all the time. When you're not on top form, choose a perfume to lift your spirits. For dull, lifeless skin use orchid or mandarin flower scents. To make you feel super-sophisticated use clementine. It's well known that a happy woman is a beautiful woman.

● ● ● DID YOU KNOW?

> Laughter is the best medicine for chasing away a dull expression. Think of it as interior jogging. When you laugh your heart beats as fast as if you were running 100 metres. This lowers blood pressure, improves digestion and ensures a good night's sleep.

KEY FACTS

* Good humour goes hand-in-hand with beautiful skin.

* Use perfumes which make life seem rosy.

* Don't forget to have fun. Happy women have healthy complexions.

case study

'I've never been one to spend hours over my appearance, so my beauty routine is fairly basic: I cleanse morning and night with a soap-based cream and a hydrating cream. My job is quite demanding and requires a lot of travel, as I'm Director of Marketing for an international company. Luckily I've got normal skin so I don't get too many problems. I use a two-stage solution on my eyes which is ideal for removing waterproof mascara. In the morning I always make sure I drink a long glass of water as soon as I wake up, then I have a balanced breakfast and do breathing exercises. This really gives you the feeling of oxygenating yourself and is good for general health and particularly good for the skin. If I'm very tired or overworked I'll play around with food supplements to boost my spirits and my skin. I've recently discovered which plants work for me to enhance my looks and, on the rare occasions when I've got a spare moment, I'll put a few drops in the bath and enjoy the wonderful smells and the soft skin with which they leave me.'

21

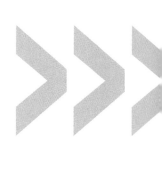

>> **Is your skin is tired, dry or oily?** Don't worry, there are a hundred and one ways to get back a healthy, balanced complexion. You just need to understand your own skin profile and learn a few tricks of the trade to make sure it's properly taken care of. Don't forget, you are unique!

>>>> **The seasons set the tone.** Exfoliate your skin in spring, gently introduce it to the summer sun, protect it from the cold in winter. There are so many thngs you can do to avoid the usual headaches.

>>>>>> **As time passes, the needs of your skin change …** so you should adjust your treatment accordingly. Discover different approaches for different problems, as and when you require them.

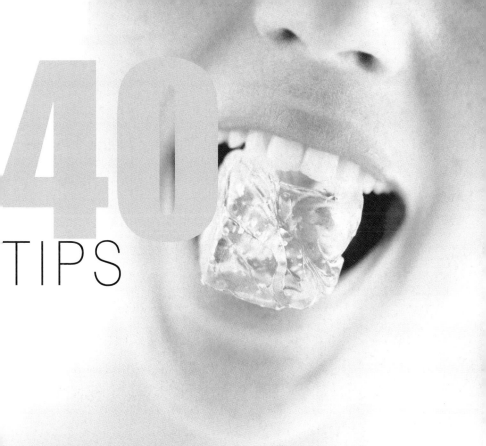

40
TIPS

21

fight fatigue

Overwork, lack of sleep, anxieties – fatigue shows in your face. There are, however, two key ways of overcoming this and giving back your skin its natural vitality. They are: improving the microcirculation and getting vitamins to the skin.

Stimulate the microcirculation

Sometimes the skin looks and feels tired and lacking in tone. This kind of fatigue is commonly attributed to our modern lifestyles and is absolutely normal. To start with, you should choose a good exfoliant which will get rid of the dead cells and improve the efficacy of the products you use afterwards. Then apply a revitalizing mask (with trace elements,

● ● ● DID YOU KNOW?

> To reduce tension and fatigue, succumb to the pleasures of a massage of the reflex zones: organize an evening of foot massage with some girlfriends. An improved complexion is guaranteed.

> Try a hydration patch. This will smooth out wrinkles, minimize fine lines and dark rings and leave your skin silky smooth.

marine concentrates and vitamins A, C and E). Used once a week, this treatment should be enough to restore your skin.

Use an energizing cream

The energy of the skin is no different from that of the body as a whole: it is maintained with the help of vitamins, fatty acids, proteins and so on. These nutrients penetrate the epidermis then go through to the dermis where they work to activate the microcirculation of the blood. Treatments which work at a surface level are therefore not always enough nor are treatments which target the interior health. The most effective are the deepest-working external treatments such as energizing creams.

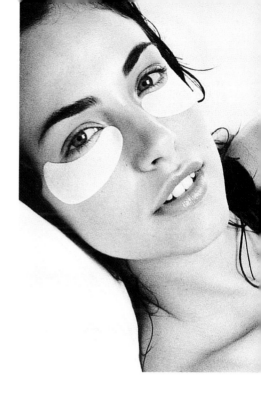

> Pay attention to your diet. Cut down on refined flour, sugar, the bad fats and products with a high milk content. Certain foods release too many toxins into the bloodstream and can drain your energy. Your skin suffers as a result.

KEY FACTS

* Take care of yourself with vitamins and a pledge of tonicity.

* Think about 'rubbing away' fatigue with an exfoliant.

* Draw strength from what you eat and eliminate foods that generate toxins.

22

calm irritated skin

If your skin is sensitive, sometimes even simple contact with water can cause irritation. There is only one answer to this: monitor your skin carefully then take action.

Identify sensitive skin

Sensitive skins sting, pull, have a tendency to redness and are prone to flaking. Any such symptom should ring alarm bells immediately. If you think about it, the skin on your face is the only part of the body, with the exception of the hands, which is always exposed to air. At the same time fragile and resistant, it reacts to the air sometimes better than other times. Certain factors such as climate change or pollution can undermine the efficacy of the skin's protective barrier. Fortunately there are skincare products especially for sensitive skin which are formulated to calm the irritation and protect against the environment. To find the ones best for you, you should, if possible, follow the advice of a pharmacist or dermatologist.

Feel comfortable in sensitive skin

Opt for products that have simple cosmetic formulas. In general, the simpler the product the better its effect. Try also to use the same cream night and morning to reduce the risk of allergic reaction. Oats and grape seed oil are the ingredients most commonly used for calming the skin.

Above all, cleanse your skin gently. Avoid products which need to be rinsed off with water.

KEY FACTS

* To reduce the risk of allergy, use the same cream day and night.

* Use a mineral water spray or vaporizer.

* Before buying a product, consult a pharmacist or dermatologist.

23

deal with dryness

How to repair a dry skin

Dry skin is highly reactive to the environment and dislikes extremes of heat, cold and wind. It tends to peel and can crease into fine surface lines. It has to be hydrated constantly.

There is a difference between a dehydrated skin and a dry skin. The one is simply thirsty, the other needs extra care in adapting a beauty regime to nourish the weakened corneal layer.

● ● ● DID YOU KNOW?

> Go back to the ancient remedies for good hydration techniques. Iris is excellent for retaining moisture in the skin, as its effect mimics the natural binding of substances in the structure of the skin.

> Drink a litre and a half (two and a half pints) of water every day to retain the hydration rate of your cells. This is as essential for your skin as it is for your overall health.

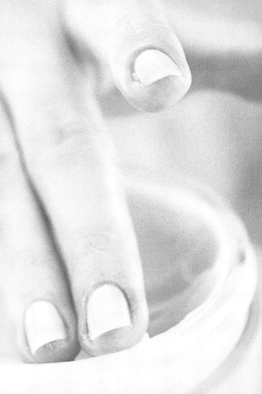

If the feeling of discomfort persists, it is essential to take action at the very first hint of trouble before the skin develops a pulling sensation. Your beauty objective should be to restore tone to the lipids in the corneal layer.

Hydrate gently

Dermatologists are unswerving in their advice: you must cleanse according to your skin type. Dry and sensitive skins need to be cleansed without removing the skin's protective film. Opt for a thick milk cleanser and rinse with flower water. Choose your cream carefully: it should be rich in repairing agents containing ceramides, which reduce the salt content and slow down the evaporation of water in the skin.

> Maximize the effects of hydration by adding the essential oil, angelica, to your day and night creams (use two drops for night time).

KEY FACTS

∗ Abandon water-based cleansers.

∗ Opt for creams with ceramides.

∗ Try iris flower and the essential oil, angelica.

24 improve your skin tone

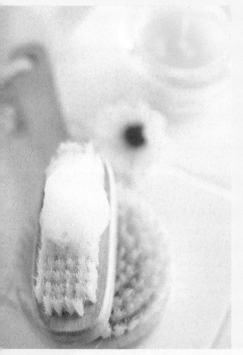

Oily skins are subject to their own particular troubles including spots, blackheads and other miseries. Excess sebum has to be controlled but today there are a number of treatments that do this effectively.

> If you use a water spray to rinse your skin, choose one rich in silica and containing derivatives of sulphur and magnesium. The latter regulate the production of sebum. Read the labels carefully before purchase.

● ● ● DID YOU KNOW?

> The salicylic acid in clay masks make them astringent. They make the skin smoother and should be applied to clean, dry skin.

Repairing oily skin

Your skin is shiny, your pores open and you often have small spots. When the sebaceous glands are overactive, the skin produces too much of the protective sebum that is lacking in dry skins. There are certain advantages to this: you are better armed to fight the ageing process and better protected against the effects of sunlight. On the other hand, your skin becomes dehydrated in the winter months and looks dull and tired. Your beauty mission is twofold – you have to absorb the excess sebum and regulate the way your skin functions.

A new routine

In order to balance oily skin, start by changing your cleansing habits. Avoid alkaline products and those containing alcohol. Wash your face with water and gentle foaming cleansers or mousses.

> Aloe vera is a great friend of oily skins; it cleanses and purifies the skin and can be purchased as a pure gel. It is also used in creams and milks.

Choose products with anti-bacterial properties that cleanse the skin thoroughly. Rinse with plenty of water, cold preferably, to close the pores.
The secret of beautiful skin resides in the pot, too. Vitamin- and mineral-based creams hydrate and rebalance in one go. Vitamin A brings a healthy glow to your skin, vitamin C fights wrinkles and zinc and magnesium control the activity of the sebaceous glands.

KEY FACTS

* Oily skins should be cleansed using water and gentle foaming cleansers.

* Choose creams rich in vitamins and minerals.

* Clay masks and aloe vera are friends of oily skin.

25

deal with combination skin

Not everybody is lucky enough to be born with a satiny skin. A large number of people suffer from dry cheeks and an oily T-zone. These are the signs of a combination skin, which requires its own particular care.

Identify a combination skin

Usually a combination skin is rough and sensitive on the cheeks where it strongly resembles dry skin. But the forehead, nose and chin areas have the tendency to shine and trap dirt common to greasy skin. Quite a tough proposition, then.

Adopt the care essentials

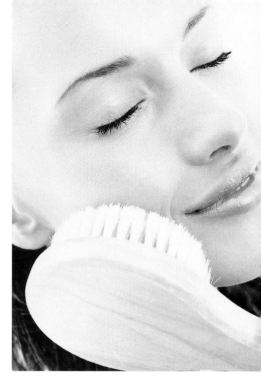

In order to avoid 'overheating' the oily areas and irritating the dry ones, you should choose a gentle cleanser. The cream cleansers which you rinse with water leave a comfortable protective layer on the skin. Apply a day cream with a high hydrating factor to the whole of your face. Blot the excess (on forehead, nose and chin) with a paper tissue.

Also available are creams specially for-mulated for combination skins which act to the improve the texture in the dry areas whilst eliminating imperfections in the T-zone. Use a matt, non-drying face powder for a peachy skin throughout the day.

> Borage can also be taken in the form of a food supplement.

KEY FACTS

* Give up using harsh soaps in favour of a more gentle cleansing cream.

* Blot the excess cream on oily areas.

* Hydrate dry areas.

* Try using borage oil.

26 minimize the effects of pollution

It is inevitable that your skin will suffer as a result of pollution, particularly if you live or work in an urban area. You can, however, incorporate specially formulated anti-pollution products, which strengthen the skin's defences, into your beauty programme.

The effects of pollution If you live in an urban environment, your skin's outer layer changes. This is because the micro-particles of pollution in the air work as oxidants. Exposed to various kinds of smoke and gases, your cells become sluggish and produce collagen of inferior quality, your skin loses its vitality, starts to sag and ages prematurely. Hence the importance of anti-pollution care.

Shield yourself from pollution The key is to find and use antioxidant substances. Vitamins A and C are the best-known sources of these and vitamin D3 is reputed to contain properties that strengthen the skin's defences. It is best to choose creams which claim to offer a 'shield' against pollution and stimulate the production of collagen. And probably your best friend of all is your regular night time cleansing ritual.

● ● ● D I D   Y O U   K N O W ?

> Try seaweed. Accustomed to put up with the diverse hazards of the sea world, the micro-organisms which it contains have developed a great facility for self-protection and regeneration. It can be found in aqua form and in the form of protective creams

K E Y   F A C T S

∗ Use creams that combat free radicals in order to protect your skin from the damaging effects of pollution.

∗ Take vitamins A, C and D3.

27 think calm

Stress is a powerful enemy of beauty. To fight it, you will have to learn to relax. To free both mind and body, take time out and allow yourself small and intermittent moments of calm and serenity.

Your skin is emotive For a long time people thought the skin was simply a kind of cover protecting the body from the outside world. How wrong they were. The skin and the brain are in fact constantly interconnected. It follows that if you feel calm your skin will look good.

Discover Japanese bathing Pamper your body the Japanese way. In the Empire of the Sun bathing is considered an important ritual for de-stressing and beautifying. Run very hot water (keep it at a constant temperature of 38°C/100°F), adding salts or perfumed effervescent bath stones. Try cedar: reminiscent of the smell of the traditional wooden bathtubs.
Play geishas with purifying kaolin masks (white clay). To soothe the skin, succumb to Japanese green-tea creams or, for a long-lasting silkiness, ginko biloba.

DID YOU KNOW?

> Incenses have a subtle influence on our behaviour. To calm your senses burn a stick of sandalwood incense or, to stay relaxed all day long, use pine: twelve minutes should be long enough for them to work their magic.

KEY FACTS

* Remember that serenity shows in the face.

* Take up Japanese beauty rituals.

* Baths, incenses and oriental massages are all highly effective ways to restore your inner calm.

28

fight
ageing

Every day the skin is involved in the process of cellular renewal. As the years pass, it loses its firmness and wrinkles appear. Remember that for all women, of any age, there are strategies you can adopt to fight ageing and hold on to your looks.

Prevention

Amazing though it may seem, you should start taking action against the ageing process at the age of 16. The first thing to do is to establish and maintain a daily cleansing and hydrating routine. This will be even more effective if you precede the application of your cream by a massage to stimulate the microcirculation.

Anti-wrinkle products are good as long as you change them from time to time over the years to adjust to the changing needs of your skin.

Anti-wrinkle strategies

Age 25 to 30: the key word is hydration. You should apply a hydrating cream morning and night. For extra radiance, alternate with a fruit acid treatment. Take special trouble with the delicate area around the eyes: this will be one of the first casualties of ageing.

Age 30 to 40: Stimulate the cells. Your skin is already asking for the anti-ageing formulas and the richer textures. Alternate with anti-fatigue treatments (vitamins and trace elements). Choose a more robust eye cream.

Age 40 to 50: Fight against slackening skin and muscles. Go for the firming creams (seaweed and ceramide) to make up for loss of collagen. Use serums and other skin-firming products.

50+ : There are special treatments available for use during the menopause specially adapted to the hormone changes in your body.

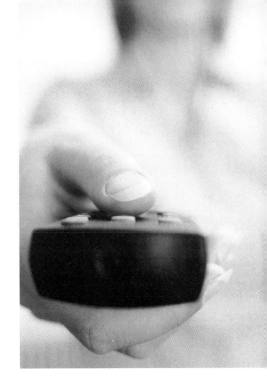

KEY FACTS

* Start with a preventative beauty care regime from the age of 16.

* Adapt your anti-age treatments according to your age group.

* Protect your skin from free radicals (cigarette smoke, sun, pollution) which all contribute to premature ageing.

29

stay young

It doesn't matter how old you are: beauty doesn't disappear at the first sign of wrinkles. But, it is up to you to have a lifestyle that is kind to your skin. Certain anti-age treatments can also give you a feeling of all-round rejuvenation.

Maintain a healthy lifestyle

You can make yourself feel young in a number of ways. For a start, try to avoid situations which encourage faster ageing of the cells, such as too much exposure to the sun, pollution and stress. As far as wrinkles go, a healthy lifestyle is an excellent antidote: have lots of rest, eat a balanced diet and drink plenty of water.

● ● ● DID YOU KNOW?

> You can find plant-based anti-ageing products at most pharmacies. Borage oil, for example, is rich in the unsaturated fatty acids devoured by the skin (in tablet form you should take it for a period of a month at a time).

> Vitamins – notably A, C and E, are also important in the fight against ageing. Try to get them in their most natural forms for a month at a time. And don't forget to eat plenty of fresh fruit and vegetables.

Zoom in on retinol

Retinol is a high-performance anti-wrinkle treatment. An alcoholic form of vitamin A, it greatly improves hydration and gives back the skin its suppleness and elasticity. There are a range of enticing retinol creams and serums on the market today. Use them together with fruit acids to lift and restore your beauty. Certain creams also contain retinaldehyde, which aids the cells to secrete natural retinol. For best results, use for one to two months.

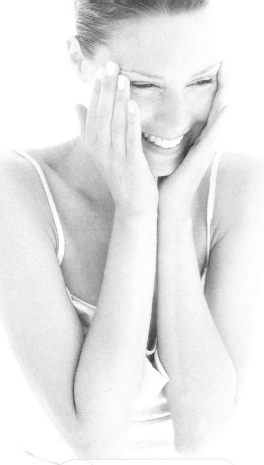

> The lifting effect: experiment with serums based on plant extracts. Massage into the skin once a day in the early evening. Continue for a month.

KEY FACTS

* Give your face back its radiance with a healthy lifestyle.

* Speed up cellular renewal with retinol.

* Fill up with vitamins.

30

find that healthy glow again

Deep purifying is a great way of giving the skin back its luminosity and can be done from time to time to boost everyday cleansing. It will get rid of all those dead cells and give you a squeaky-clean complexion.

Get rid of impurities

The skin loses its cool over the smallest things. A liitle fatigue, a polluted atmosphere... but there are certain measures you can take to get your skin back to tip-top form and cleanliness. The key is to get rid of the dead cells so that treatment creams can better nourish the new cells. You can use deep-penetrating treatments – natural marine acid or fruit acid peeling, for example; or you can use that ancient and ultra-natural method: the facial sauna.

Have a facial sauna

The sauna is an excellent way to deep-cleanse the skin. The steam gently dilates the pores and lifts out toxins, leaving your skin polished.
• Fill a bowl with a litre (about two pints) of boiling water. Add three drops of essential oils (bergamot or lemon for oily skin, camomile or neroli for dry skin, lavender or rose for sensitive skin, sandalwood or rosemary for wrinkles).
• Place the bowl so that you can lean forward to it from a sitting position without discomfort.
• Put a towel over your head, bend over the bowl and make sure that the towel fully covers your head and the bowl. Remove after 10 minutes.
• Spray your face with fresh water from an atomizer to retighten the pores.
• Dry gently without rubbing, then apply a rich hydrating cream.
• Your skin will now be bright and squeaky-clean.

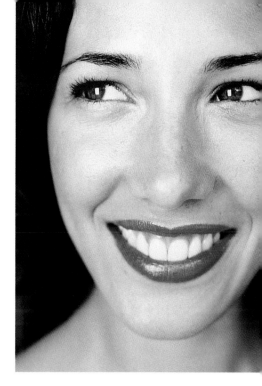

KEY FACTS

* Remove dead cells in order to renew your skin.

* Have a facial sauna and you will see a huge difference in skin clarity.

* Boost your cells with vitamins to counteract fatigue.

31

be radiant every day, every month

We all know that our periods affect our skin just as they do much as our moods. Shiny skin, a drawn look... and your regular treatment doesn't help. But cheer up – there are ways to be radiant every day, every month.

Did you say hormones?

When you have your period your body is depleted of energy, making you feel tired and down, and often giving you a drawn look. This is in fact caused by a hormonal imbalance. The hormones prepare the body for pregnancy throughout the monthly cycle, releasing more oestrogen in the first two weeks and more progesterone in the last two weeks. The days in the middle when the hormones levels are switching, and the days of the period itself are when your skin is most vulnerable, and it is at these times you should take extra special care of it.

Think plants

• **The skin on your cheeks and around the eyes may appear stretched or pulled.** If this is the case, apply a hydrating mask to irrigate and retain surface water.

- **For shininess on the wings of the nose,** use an absorbent clay mask.
- **If you have an outbreak of spots,** after cleansing you should apply a cotton bud dipped in lavender oil directly onto them. Lavender is a natural disinfectant and astringent and is one of the rare essential oils which can be used on the skin with no risk of reaction.
- **Drink herbal teas** which can help your body at this difficult time: fennel, sage and camomile.

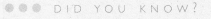

DID YOU KNOW?

> Latent health problems often come out into the open when you have your period. This does not help the complexion and can give you dark rings under the eyes. To counteract this you must relax. Lie down comfortably, loosen your shoulders and keep your head straight to allow a free blood flow from the vertebral column. Close your eyes. Try to be aware of your breathing: fill your stomach with air on breathing in, then breathe out deeply. Say to yourself, 'I accept the changes in my body and I can help myself feel better.'

KEY FACTS

* The hormonal changes brought about by the menstrual cycle upset the balance of the skin.

* Take herbal teas for your complexion and essential oils for outbreaks of spots.

32

banish
puffy eyes

Puffy eyelids, dark rings, wrinkles...the eye contour is often the place where the first signs of ageing are visible. The skin around the eyes is very fine and therefore highly delicate. The best way to take care of it is to combine special treatments with a healthy lifestyle.

Eye care

The delicate area around the eye is prone to certain specific problems. When you wake up in the morning you will often see the signs of these, such as under-eye bags, protein deposits and little localized swellings. Ageing only adds to the likelihood of developing problems, causing as it does a slow-down in the microcirculation. To take daily care of the eye area start by giving up smoking as the nicotine intake further slows down the production of collagen. Get enough sleep: this is still the best way to ensure you have sparkling eyes. Finally, drink a large glass of water at night before going to sleep and one in the morning as soon as you wake up. This will help to eliminate the toxins which drain into the eyelids when you are sleeping for several hours.

Relieve congestion

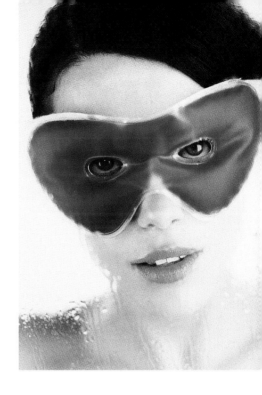

For no more puffy eyes when you wake up, splash thermal water on you face for at least 30 seconds. Studies have shown this has a soothing effect on the eyes. To refresh them further, try a cooling gel eye mask straight from the refrigerator. This is also good when you have red or watery eyes. You can also use a firming serum around the eyes, or you can use specialist eye drops to relieve congestion and flush out excess water (available from most pharmacies).

> Use cornflower water (eau de bleuet). Containing astringent and anti-inflammatory properties, it has a pleasant calming effect on sore eyelids. Put a few drops on some cotton wool and place over your eyes.

KEY FACTS

* The area around the eyes is one of the most delicate in the body because the skin is so fine there.

* Stop smoking, bathe your eyes with thermal water on waking up and use herbal tea compresses.

33

detox in the spring

At the first sign of spring your skin will start demanding a particular kind of care. It's time to scrub away the winter months, refresh and rejuvenate your skin and work out a detox programme.

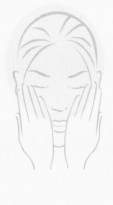
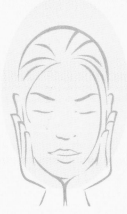

Spring-clean your body

In spring your body needs to be drained of all the toxins accumulated during winter (such as lactic and uric acid). This means reinvigorating the eliminatory organs – liver, kidneys, lungs and skin. The best treatments are the most natural ones: plants, fruit juices or vegetables. Fennel in particular helps the kidneys get rid of water. Black radishes and artichoke are good for the liver, whilst mallow and marshmallow stimulate the intestines. Burdock purifies the skin.

It's good to drain

To drain your face, remove all make-up and cleanse thoroughly. Then apply a gentle, circular palm massage positioning the hands as follows:
• **Cheeks:** put your hands on your cheeks above the side of the nose. Hold this position for 10 to 15 seconds.

- **Chin and facial contour:** rest your chin in the palms of your hands which should be joined together at the wrists. Enclose the oval of your face in your hands. Hold this position for 10 to 15 seconds.
- **Ears:** place your hands at the base of your ears. Hold the position for around 10 seconds.

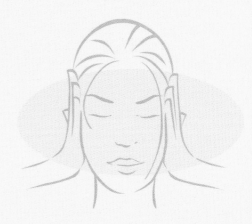

● ● ● DID YOU KNOW?

> To detoxify your body, try clay milk (see Tip 33). Put a spoonful of clay into a glass of water and leave overnight, drinking it the next morning. Continue every night and morning for two weeks. Make sure you use a good quality clay and a lightly mineralized water. If you can face it, stir the liquid with a wooden spoon before drinking: it's more effective to drink the clay at the same time as the water. Otherwise just drink the water; the clay absorbs the impurities and gently helps you get rid of them.

KEY FACTS

* It is important to drain the impurities from the body in spring.

* Take a plant cure to help your body get rid of toxins.

* Try a course of lymphatic drainage for your face.

34 benefit from the sun

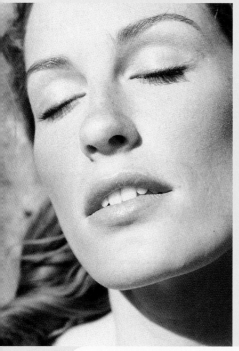

Sunshine is the source of all life and is the key to healthy good looks. But be careful. As far as your skin goes, it can also be enemy number one. It is vital to know how to benefit from the sun without the risk of damage.

DID YOU KNOW?

> You can also help protect your skin using plants:

> Before a tanning session take horsetail. It is rich in vitamins, notably silicon, which exists naturally in the cutaneous tissue. Use it in the form of capsules, herbal teas or fresh in salads.

Sun tolerance

We don't all react the same way to sun exposure. Your body can tolerate more or less sun depending on your skin type. If you have dark hair and eyes and matt skin then you should have a naturally higher sun tolerance factor than a blonde with blue eyes. But the more you expose your skin to the sun, the more vulnerable it becomes. To protect itself the skin produces melanine, which is also what gives you your tan. Some people produce more melanine than others; some produce better quality melanine than others. The key to safe and better tanning is to stimulate the production of melanine.

Tyrosine and vitamins

Certain creams contain natural melanine-enhancing properties such as tyrosine. You should begin to use them twelve days before exposure to the sun and take plenty of vitamins. The three antioxidant vitamins A, C and E form a barrier against the increased production of free radicals by the solar rays. If your general intake of fruit and vegetables is low, increase your consumption for a month or so before you go to the sun. You can also take a beta-carotene supplement: this will tan the skin lightly and increase your sun tolerance.

KEY FACTS

* Protect your skin according to your personal sun-tolerance factor.

* Tyrosine stimulates the production of melanine.

* Take plenty of antioxidant vitamins and beta-carotene.

* Take horsetail and rosemary before going into the sun.

> Rosemary is a good antioxidant and counteracts the dehydrating effect on the skin of the oxidization of fatty acids.

35

In recent years a lot of research has been done on tanning and the effects of ultraviolet rays on the skin. This is invaluable in determining your individual needs and so enables you to plan a safe tanning programme.

protect yourself against UV rays

UVA and UVB

Essentially the sun gives off two types of rays: infrared, which burn and cause sunstroke; and ultraviolet, which penetrate the cutaneous barrier. The UVB rays (of average frequency) activate the melanocytes which are responsible for the production of melanine, and slowly but surely bronze the skin. The UVA rays however (which are of a higher frequency) penetrate right through to the cells, damaging them and causing premature ageing and skin cancers. The idea then is to choose products which will protect the skin from the harmful solar rays whilst not blocking the beneficial ones.

High protection factors

Sun creams come with different protection factors indicating strength in filtering the harmful solar rays. The higher the number the greater the protection. For the first few days in the sun everyone should use a high protection-factor cream. After that the choice of sun-protection factor will depend on skin type.

Blondes and redheads with fair skins should not go lower than factor 30. If you have brown hair with a medium skin tone you can go down to factor 20 after the first week. People with dark hair and olive skin can use factor 15 or even 10 after three or four days providing the sun cream is reapplied regularly.

In all cases, dermatologists advise that sun exposure should be before noon and after 4-5pm, and must be very gradual. Do 15 minutes the first day, adding ten minutes daily until reaching the maximum exposure time for your skin type, with two hours being the longest even the most sun resistant should stay in the sun.

● ● ● DID YOU KNOW?

> For enjoyable sun-lounging with wrinkle-free tanning, increase your vitamin consumption in the foods you eat. Summer is the ideal season for fresh fruit and vegetables, either lightly cooked or raw. Artichokes, aubergines/egg plants, celery, broccoli and spinach are all good because they are rich in zinc, silicon and vitamin C, and hydrate the skin from the inside. To speed up tanning, eat fruits and vegetables of an orange colour, high in beta-carotene, such as carrots, melon, apricots and peaches.

KEY FACTS

* To tan without giving yourself wrinkles, change your diet.

* Follow sun-protection factor guides carefully.

* Make sure you build up sun exposure gradually and never sunbathe at the hottest time of the day.

36

stay bronzed

Everybody wants a beautiful, long-lasting, even tan. The good news is that it can be achieved by combining a good pre- and during -tanning regime with appropriate after-sun care.

Maintain the skin's hydration rate

Prolonged exposure to the sun sets off real molecular changes that the skin has to spend several days repairing. Dehydration and production of poor-quality collagen are just two of the effects. To prevent these problems get into good habits during and after tanning. Doing this will protect your skin from damage and ensure a lasting colour.

● ● ● DID YOU KNOW?

> In summer the skin is exposed to hot, dry air, salt from the beach and the sea and the chlorine from swimming pools. Remember to look after your skin from the inside as well as the outside.

> Vitamin and mineral capsules which prepare the skin for tanning also prolong the life of your tan. Continue your course for two or three weeks after your return from holiday.

When you leave the beach, always take a shower then dry yourself without rubbing and apply an after-sun milk on your body. Your face will need a stronger after-sun treatment, such as an ampule of serum.

Avoid peeling

To prolong your tan once you have returned from your holiday it is essential to avoid peeling, which is the loss of cells through dryness. A light exfoliation once or twice a week will get rid of dead cells whilst not damaging the rest. It's true that your tan will fade a little, but it will be more even and your skin will appear much clearer.

Continue your after-sun care for face and body for several weeks after your holiday. This will gradually replenish lost water and restructure the skin, making it more supple and giving it a healthy glow. Above all, do not skimp on the use of an ultra-hydrating cream which is both repairing and antioxidant. If you have oily or combination skin, choose one with aloe; for normal or dry skin, select one with shea tree butter.

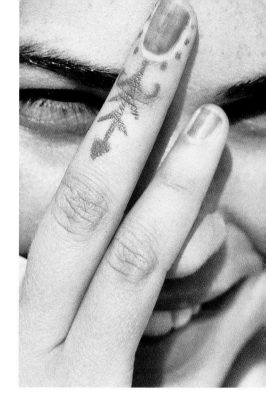

 KEY FACTS

∗ To keep your tan you need to take steps to avoid peeling.

∗ A light exfoliation evens the skin tone and prolongs your tan.

∗ Continue after-sun care for several weeks to ensure a long-lasting colour.

Certain parts of the body – particularly the hands and the lips – are more sensitive to the cold than others. It's essential to start taking extra care of these areas straight away at the onset of winter.

Lips are fragile The lips are extremely delicate with a very fine corneal layer and high vein content. The skin of the lips is ultra-thin and does not contain any sebum, which means that they have no natural protection from cold and dryness. To avoid chapped lips it is essential to apply a hydrating balm at regular intervals. The best ones are those containing natural ingredients: honey, grapefruit, plant extracts etc.

Your hands need you Your hands take a lot of wear and are in frequent contact with harmful substances such as detergents and hard water. Without protection they will suffer horribly in the cold. In the winter, more than any other time, you should use a hand cream, preferably several times a day. The ones with silicone, honey or lanolin protect the skin whilst the ones with shea tree butter or glycerine nourish the skin. After you wash your hands always be sure to dry them thoroughly before applying the cream.

● ● ● D I D   Y O U   K N O W ?

> Moistening the lips with saliva only aggravates the dryness.

> The best time to repair the damage done by the cold is during the night. Before going to bed put a generous layer of hand cream onto your hands, then slip on a pair of cotton gloves.

KEY FACTS

* Protect your lips with a balm containing natural ingredients.

* Apply hand cream several times a day.

38 give up smoking

Smoking, as everyone knows, is detrimental for our health. It is also an enemy of the skin as it speeds up the appearance of wrinkles. To recognize it as such is the first step towards finding an antidote.

Tobacco and oxygen The oxygen content of the skin decreases with age. So too does its softness and elasticity. Smoking does nothing at all to help: with the intake of nicotine the epidermis gets thinner, the elastin slackens and the skin dehydrates, whilst the tar in cigarettes multiplies the production of free radicals which cause ageing.

Only one answer There is only one answer: give up smoking. Of course this is usually a lot easier said than done. No technique is going to work that well if you haven't truly taken the decision to stop. If you are ready to give up, then there are a range of methods you can try: patches, acupuncture, homeopathy, plants, auriculotherapy, psychotherapy, group counselling and so on.

● ● ● DID YOU KNOW?

> If you do smoke, try using an oxygenating cream, which will help your skin breathe and brighten the complexion. It is also advisable for non-smokers who live or work in a smoky atmosphere.

KEY FACTS

* Stop smoking. Tobacco suffocates the skin.

* Help yourself by trying acupuncture, homeopathy, support groups etc.

* Use an oxygenating cream on your skin.

39 be ready for the cold months

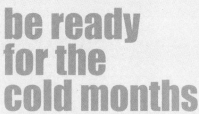

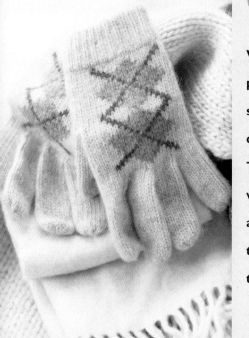

When the temperature drops skin problems soar. No matter what your skin type, you will experience some degree of dryness and dehydration. This is because the protective film which covers the skin is no longer fully able to carry out its function against the environmental aggressions. So, take action at the first signs of trouble.

> To guard against nutrition deficiencies which can cause excessive dryness and loss of elasticity, include as many essential fatty acids in your food as possible: eat oily fish such as salmon and herring, vegetable oils, nuts (especially almonds and hazelnuts) and dry fruits. These fatty acids

Fight the frost

The skin doesn't like bad weather. Wind, rain and cold are real problems for it as the lipids which form the protective barrier in the corneal layer are less efficient. Sudden changes in the weather are also bad for the skin: going from cold to hot or from hot to cold encourages the little red veins on the cheek and nose to dilate. It's important to act quickly when the first signs of sensitivity appear. Gingko biloba, in the form of capsules or creams, is great for repairing the elasticity of the capillaries.

Warm winter woollies

Once again dehydration is the biggest threat to your skin in cold weather conditions. This happens when the lipids in the intercellular cement which provide the cellular cohesion begin to disperse.

are the basic components of the epidermis and stop the skin from cracking in the cold weather. You can also take them in capsule form for a minimum three-month period.
> To stop red blotches in their tracks, use creams containing ruscus, butcher's broom or horse chestnut which decongest the skin without irritating it.

Don't think twice about buying a cream for very dry skin, such as a cold cream, low in water but high in oil content. It will deposit hydrating agents on the skin's surface and leave a light protective film. In winter you get out your heavy woolly clothes, so do the same for your skin. Use natural oils (jojoba, wheatgerm, for example) to reinforce the effects of your protective day or night cream.

KEY FACTS

* In very cold weather conditions use a cold cream or a cream for very dry skin.

* Include essential fatty acids in your diet (oily fish, vegetable oils and dried fruits).

* Horse chestnut, butcher's broom and ginko biloba work well against redness in sensitive skins.

40 prolong youthfulness

Defy the passing years with a hand massage. Using a combination of manual techniques and advanced technology, you can prolong youthfulness.

The face-lift massage: of the anti-ageing treatments and techniques, the massage has certainly proved its worth. Treat yourself to a face-lift massage once a month in a salon, or do your own treatment in the bath or after a face mask.

Get that glow

Forehead: place your thumbs in the centre of your forehead. Move in a circular motion going outwards towards the temples. Repeat three times. Finish by pressing the centre of the temples.

Nose: using small circular movements, massage the wings of the nose, from the bottom of the eyebrows to the base of the nose. Then repeat in the opposite direction starting from the base of the nose. Repeat six times.

Mouth: with the index and middle fingers of each hand, apply a gentle pressure along the lower lip starting at the centre and moving outwards. Repeat six times.

KEY FACTS

* Put your trust in a manual face massage.

* Learn how to do a home massage.

* Go technological with ionization.

case study

I'm a dab hand with a spring cure

'Every spring, without fail, I have the same problem: my skin looks dull and I get spots. One year I'd had enough and decided to consult a dermatologist. He prescribed a treatment which helps my body to get rid of the winter toxins. Now, from the end of March, I take this treatment which consists of various draining, purifying plants: fennel, orthosiphon, black radish, burdock....The effect is radical: my complexion is clearer, my skin can breathe better and by eating healthily I can increase this effect even further. Lots of fresh fruit and vegetables, dried fruits, oily fish and raw vegetable oils, plus food supplements containing yeast for their B vitamins. As I have to stand for the whole morning at work (I'm a hostess employed by a company to welcome clients) I've also got into the habit of having lymphatic drainage to improve my blood and lymphatic circulation. I pamper myself every so often by booking in to a beauty salon, which makes me feel wonderful. If I had my way I'd go once a week!'

41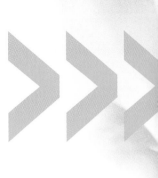

>> **Red blotches, dark rings, acne?** The skin can be a depressing variety of colours. To overcome these problems, try to work out what lies at the source of the condition.

>>>> **Skin problems can be solved,** you just need to learn to control them. If, for example, your skin reacts badly to weather conditions, you can find out which natural treatments to use to prevent and treat these problems.

>>>>>> **It's important to have a positive and healthy outlook.** The skin is a mirror of the emotions. You can improve your interior and exterior health simultaneously with homeopathy, psychotherapy or thalassotherapy. Follow our advice and don't hesitate to consult a specialist if your skin problems are chronic.

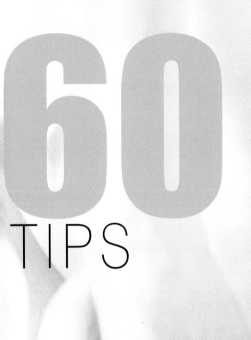

60
TIPS

Nature is incredible providing us, as she does, with a multitude of plants that heal cuts, bruises and burns thanks to their repairing and regenerating properties.

41
use healing
plant extracts

Arnica, the bruise-buster

Arnica has long been known for its healing action on bruises. If on waking tomorrow morning you sit up suddenly and hit your forehead on the cupboard door, your best bet will be arnica. You could of course cover the bruise with foundation or a concealer but that is not the quickest way to get rid of it. Arnica is effective because it disperses the build-up of blood in the damaged tissues.

● ● ● DID YOU KNOW?

> Wild horsetail, rich in minerals and particularly in silicon, is highly effective in repairing the cutaneous tissues.

> Horsetail stimulates the production of collagen and has a direct action on the conjunctive tissue. Buy a pot of it to make into herbal tea. Use 30g (1½ oz) for every litre (1¾ pints) of water, boiling for 10 minutes. Drink between 250 and 500ml (8 and 17fl oz) per day.

Mix 1 spoonful of arnica powder with nine spoonfuls of mineral water and apply as a compress to the affected area.

For injuries, calendula

Like arnica, calendula has been known for centuries for its healing properties. This humble garden herb works wonders for minor cuts and skin irritations. It is mild enough to be used on all skins, even a baby's. Containing allantoin, amino acids and beta- carotene, it is a natural regenerator that speeds up the reconstruction of the outer layer of skin. Apply the powder as a compress directly to the wound (dilution 1/10), or use in cream form to soothe the skin after shaving or in cold weather conditions. Calendula oil, in combination with aloe gel, can be used to treat eczema.

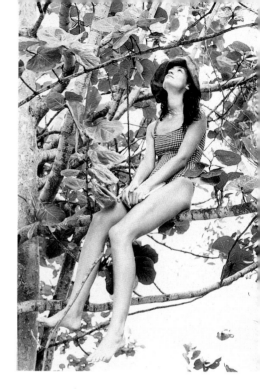

KEY FACTS

* Calendula is the king of healing. It also is good for calming irritated skin.

* Arnica compresses are effective in the treatment of bruises.

* Horsetail is renowned for its regenerative properties.

42

meet the fumitory herb

Fumitory is a plant of African origin which has been used for over a thousand years by the Arab people in the treatment of skin complaints (particularly sores). As a herbal drink or a compress, it works as a purgative and a pick-me-up.

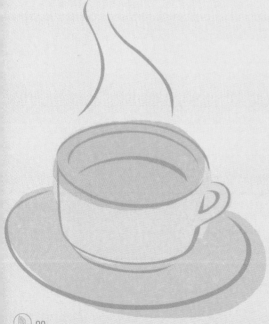

More about the herb

Fumitory is a truly extraordinary herb, containing as it does many effective properties. Its purgative action has been known since ancient times when the Arab women traditionally used it for refining the complexion. Nowadays its most popular use is in the treatment of sores, particularly for those found around the mouth area which tend to appear in winter with the cold weather. Stress and fatigue can also cause these sores which are annoying and demoralizing though not generally itchy.

Enthuse about infusions

Take fumitory internally in the form of a herbal infusion for eight days (maximum). Using the airy parts of the plant (leaves and flowers) mix 1 level teaspoon into a cup of boiling water and leave to stand for 10 minutes before drinking. Take 3 times daily without food. You can also add burdock root and walnut leaves to the infusion which may speed up the healing process. If the skin complaint persists, consult a doctor.

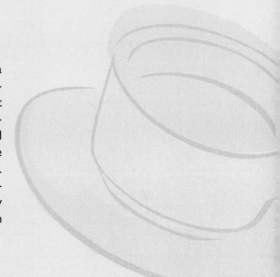

● ● ● D I D Y O U K N O W ?

> Clay is excellent for removing impurities and replacing minerals in the skin. Try making up some clay milk (see Tip 33).

> For localized irritations, apply compresses of evening primrose oil or borage oil. These can calm the skin using a deep penetrating action.

> Use a rich treatment cream with a long-lasting oil ingredient.

KEY FACTS

* The purgative properties of fumitory are highly effective in the treatment of sores.

* Drink 3 cups of fumitory tea every day for 8 days.

* Give yourself a regular clay treatment.

43 deal with rosacea

A little rosy glow on the cheeks can be attractive but permanent redness is less so. The risk of blotchy skin or rosacea may be lurking and you need to watch out for it. Happily, there are treatments that can deal with the condition and return your skin to a youthful radiance.

within the skin. Only electrodessication or laser treatment can remove them permanently.

Handle with care

It starts with a redness that comes to your cheeks at the slightest hint of emotion. Going bright red is an early sign of rosacea. Broken capillaries become fragile due to a sluggish movement in the veins of your face and if you don't do something about it, the vessels may burst, leaving your cheeks permanently red. This condition is rosacea and it can affect the network of blood vessels in your outer layer of skin.

You need to limit the loss of water from the epidermis and reinforce the elasticity of the capillaries.

Combat redness

You should cleanse with gentle products. Creamy cleansers or milky make-up removers are recommended.

Avoid water that is too warm and try sprays of mineral water instead. Always dry your skin carefully.

> Take preventive action - avoid major changes in temperature, such as going out in the snow or enjoying Turkish baths. Give up smoking and avoid spicy food and alcohol.

Protect your cheeks with creams that combat redness. Most effective in the long terms are those containing plant extracts – ivy, vine, ginkgo biloba and horse chestnut. These plants strengthen the venous walls and improve blood circulation. Massage a small amount of cream into your face, morning and night, using a gentle circular motion.

KEY FACTS

* Rosacea results from fragile, broken capillary vessels in the face.

* Use plant-based creams containing horse chestnut, ivy and gingko biloba.

* You may have to resort to laser treatment to remove the condition.

44

Warts are most commonly found on the hands but they also appear on the face and neck. Though they are extremely unattractive they are persistent and difficult to treat and a lot of people simply don't bother to treat them. The most effective remedies are plants and homeopathy.

wage war on warts

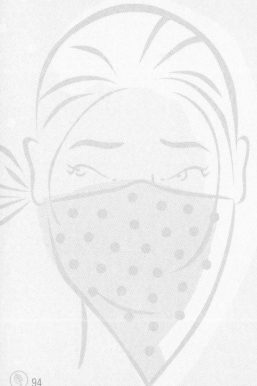

Don't ignore your warts

Warts are small growths which appear and disappear for no apparent reason. They are often caused by psychological factors. Caused by the paillomavirus (HPV), they are not a serious health problem but are nonetheless unpleasant particularly when situated on the eyelids, face or neck. They tend to last several months and may be quite numerous. Only in severe cases when they are large and multiple are they associated with immune deficiency.

Try homeopathy

Homeopathy can take a long time to work and requires patience but if you persist your patience should be rewarded. The remedies recommended are prescribed according to the type of wart and where it is on the body.

• For all treatments: take one dose of thuja 15 C, three times per day, on alternate weeks.

• For large or painful warts on the feet or hands: take *Antimonium crudum* 9 C.
• For yellowish warts where there is bleeding: take *Nitricum acidum* 9 C.
• Warts around the nail areas: take *Graphites* 9 C.
• Flat warts on the hands especially on fingertips: take *Berberis* 9 C.

KEY FACTS

* Homeopathy is the best way to get rid of warts.

* Choose the remedy according to the type of wart and where it is localized.

* Use thuja and chelidonium lotion.

45

say goodbye
to herpes

Herpes is a virus which appears most frequently in the summer months. Sun is a trigger. It appears on the mouth in the form of grouped blisters on a red base. One way of treating herpes is with plant extracts. First of all be sure to diagnose herpes correctly before treatment.

Identify the intruder

Herpes starts with a tingling sensation then it gets itchy. Next a red patch will appear followed by a blister on the edge of the lip, which then erupts.

In fact the herpes virus (*herpes hominis*) lies dormant in the vast majority of people. It breaks out when your immune system is more than usually vulnerable.

● ● ● DID YOU KNOW?

> Try oligotherapy: copper (or the copper-magnesium duo) dissolved on the tongue, is good remedy for boosting a weakened immune system.

> Change your diet to prevent the re-occurrence of the virus. Avoid almonds, walnuts and hazelnuts and increase your intake of meat and soya: the lysine in them can stop herpes emerging.

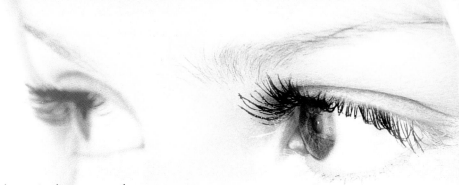

A change in diet, too much sun, stress, fever, tiredness can all precipitate an outbreak. Herpes usually appears on the mouth but can also occur on the eyelids and in the genital area. Be careful, because it is highly contagious and can be spread by only the briefest contact.

Discover phytotherapy

Echinacea is a small plant which boasts large pink flowers and remarkable anti-herpetic properties. It both cures and prevents outbreaks. It works by stimu-lating the immune system thereby enabling the body to protect itself against infection. Its efficacy has been shown by numerous pharmacological studies. If you are prone to herpes, use it as a preventative at times when you are likely to be vulnerable, such as changes of season or going off on holiday. It is available in various forms, for both inter-nal and external use: in a powder, in capsules, pomade and cream.

KEY FACTS

* Echinacea is very effective in treating outbreaks of herpes.

* Take copper and magnesium.

* To prevent a further outbreak, eat foods rich in lysine.

Acne is probably one of the most distressing skin problems. It generally occurs during adolescence although older people can also be affected. Caused by an imbalance in the sebaceous secretions, a rigorous cleansing programme and plant-based treatments can considerably improve matters.

46
treat acne

Adolescent blues

Acne is one of the miseries of adolescence. Generally thought of as a benign skin problem, it can have long-term consequences. It manifests itself in blocking and inflammation of the sebaceous follicle with the formation of blackheads, whiteheads, inflamed papules and pustules, and small facial spots can become infected. Common treatments from your doctor include antibiotics and topical agents that

> Certain plant-based treatments drain the toxins found in skin with acne. Burdock purifies the blood and speeds up the elimination of metabolic waste. To alternate, use wild pansy every other week which has superb purifying and healing properties. Dandelion stimulates the liver and encourages the secretions of bile. Take it in the form of capsules or herbal tea.

encourage unblocking of the pilosebaceous units. Derivations of vitamin A are available as creams and lotions. For severe acne powerful retinoids and vitamin A can be taken orally. They are available on prescription only due to their side effects.

Treating acne

A skin which has acne is by definition an oily skin, so follow the same daily care programme as that recommended for oily skins. In addition, clean the skin thoroughly with a dermatological glycerine soap containing antibacterial agents. Skin suffering from acne is often irritated by over-drying from oily skin treatments. In this case it is preferable to use an emulsion-based day cream (oil in water) containing zinc gluconate and emollients. Other types of emulsion, unscented, containing zinc salts and allantoin have the advantage of being thick in texture with easy absorption into the skin.

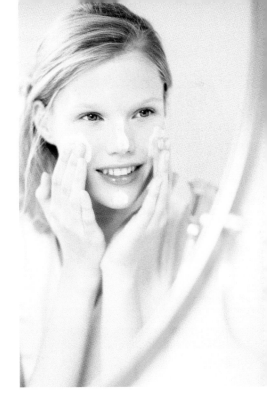

➤ Ask your pharmacist to make up the following solution: 30 drops each of the essential oils of lavender, oregano and thyme mixed with 125ml (4fl oz) sweet almond oil. Apply externally.

KEY FACTS

* Clean your skin with a bar of dermatological soap.

* Drain your body of toxins with plants: burdock, dandelion and wild pansy.

* Apply a solution of essential oils to affected areas.

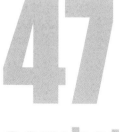

47

combat
psoriasis

People who suffer from psoriasis can sometimes feel like social outcasts. Their skin flakes and peels dramatically and tends to get inflamed. Yet with a healthy lifestyle and appropriate dermatological care, it is possible to ameliorate this skin disorder.

Focus on psoriasis

Though less common than eczema, psoriasis nonetheless affects 2.5% of the population. This skin disorder takes the form of red patches covered with a white layer of dead cells (scales). It tend to favour the elbows, knees, scalp and the creases of the buttocks. Normall the epidermis renews itself once ever 28 days. With psoriasis this process is se back by 5 to 7 days. As a result the skin

● ● ● DID YOU KNOW?

> There are various homeopathic treatments for psoriasis:
> If you are depressed, and the psoriasis is in the folds of the skin or around the nail area, try Sepia 5 C.

> If you suffer from anxiety, require constant reassurance and are prone to exhaustion, take Phosphorus 5 C.

peels and gets inflamed. This problem can become chronic. Psoriasis tends to run in families and can be triggered by streptococcal throat infections, some medicines, UV light, stress and alcohol.

Hydrotherapy can help

The success of the treatment for psoriasis depends on several factors. We know that thermal springs inhibit the regeneration of the allergic cells, reduce inflammation and have a positive antioxidant effect. The key to the treatment is in the bathing itself. Other treatments, such as facial or general body sprays, work to soften the skin whilst reducing irritation. Finally, the cure can lie simply in coming to terms with the affliction and making an effort to socialize despite your inhibitions. Psoriasis is often a psychosomatic illness and may be aggravated by stress.

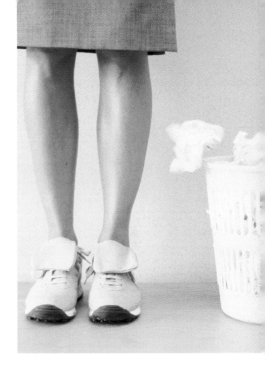

> If you are fastidious by nature, or are afraid of growing old: try *Arsenicum album*.
> Take all the above remedies doses of 3 granules night and morning for a month.

  KEY FACTS

* Take a thermal cure: the water inhibits the multiplication of the cells which cause psoriasis.

* Go out socially: psychological support is one way of helping to get better.

* For a gentle and effective treatment try homeopathy.

48

Brown marks, the mask of pregnancy, and stretch marks are all part of pregnancy and can be remedied by natural methods. Don't worry, you can boast a round tummy and a radiant complexion at the same time.

be beautiful in pregnancy

Pregnancy alters the nature of your skin

When you are pregnant, your body changes dramatically. Hormones released during pregnancy transform the nature of your skin, and the secretion of oil from the sebaceous glands may increase or decrease. Signs of fatigue appear when you look in the mirror. It's time to pamper your skin. Firstly, exfoliate to remove all dead skin and then cleanse and tone to remove excess grease and control shine. If, however, your skin feels tight, use a hydrating mask. If brownish or yellowish marks appear on your face, don't panic! Chloasma, otherwise known as the mask of pregnancy, usually disappears after you have given birth. In any case, plant extracts can help reduce the visibility of the marks, in particular parsley, lime blossom, violet and heather. Enjoy them as an infusion, adding a teaspoon of each for every large bowl of boiling water. Allow to infuse and drink three cups a day.

Avoid stretch marks

If you want to wear revealing clothes after giving birth, start the battle against stretch marks early. These marks can appear on the hips, breasts and thighs from the fourth month of pregnancy and result from damage to the skin's elasticity. Once this rupture occurs, the fibres don't fully repair. Prevention is the answer as there is no cure.

Try to apply a specific cream to combat stretch marks every day. Some contain gentle, nourishing sweet almond oil which moisturizes the skin deeply. Others are silicon-based and stimulate the fibroblasts. Creams containing trace elements help produce high quality collagen. Spend at least five minutes a day massaging your skin with the cream.

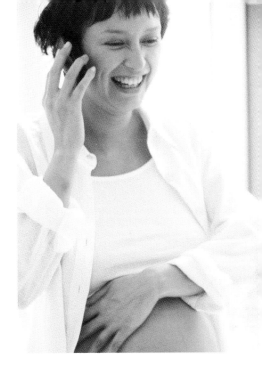

KEY FACTS

* Drink herbal infusions to avoid discolouration of the skin.

* Avoid stretch marks with creams containing silicon and trace elements.

* Have a massage to help you on both the emotional and physical levels.

49

talk to a psychologist

Recent studies have shown that our psychological well-being has a direct influence on the state of our skin. Sometimes your skin gives you away with its sudden outbreaks. To say goodbye to the little problems which resist the treatments of your daily beauty regime, talk to a psychologist.

Talk to your skin

The skin tells the brain what it is feeling and how its immediate environment affects it. Likewise, the brain replies. We now know that the nervous system conducts information to the skin where it is discharged in the form of biochemical substances, or neuromediators, which provoke all sorts of different reactions. It is therefore true to say that a dialogue exists between brain and skin.

Psycho-dermatological consultations

The skin is known to react violently in situations of stress, upsets or strong emotion. It gets red, inflamed, starts to itch. The neuromediators are disrupted by the excess of nervous tension. To calm things down you need to take care of the skin as well as the psyche. A psycho-dermatological consultation will address both these issues at the same time. Psychotherapy alone can also prove effective for skin problems by helping you to resolve your psychological problems.

KEY FACTS

* When you're not feeling so great, try to listen to your skin. Remember it is engaged in a permanent dialogue with your brain.

* Talk to a psychologist or a psycho-dermatologist.

* Try using Bach flower remedies.

50 deal with brown spots

Being beautiful means being in constant battle with everything that can dull your skin. Brown spots are one such adversary.

What are brown spots? Brown spots are something we could well do without. They are caused when the melanin produced by the melanocytes to protect the skin against solar rays no longer disperses, and remains blocked. However the reasons for this to happen vary. It can be down to hormonal changes (such as weight gain, a medication), ageing or excess of sun. One thing you can do to stop brown spots appearing is to protect your face in summer by using a complete sunscreen.

De-pigmenting creams Once you have got brown spots, there is only one solution, and that is to use a de-pigmenting cream. These contain substances which unblock the melanin and slow down the activity of the melanocytes. If this does not work for you, a dermatologist can prescribe a chemical treatment containing quinine, vitamin A acid and corticoid, but there are known side effects.

KEY FACTS

* Brown spots are caused by an accumulation of melanin.

* Protect your face from the sun with a total sunscreen.

* Try herbal compresses.

51 beware of sun allergies

The risks of allergy and photosensitivity are considerably increased by sun exposure. It is as well to know which elements can trigger sun allergies. Perfumes, medicines and chemical filters are at the top of the list.

The sun and perfume Whenever you wear a perfume in bright sunlight, you risk photosensitivity and an allergic reaction. This is because the alcohol contained in the perfume can raise the level of the skin's sensitivity. Perfumes contain many substances that cause a violent allergic reaction triggered by UV light, which can take the form of burning, pigmentation, skin eruptions or rashes. These are characteristically in areas exposed to the sun, such as the face.

Sun filters and medication If your skin turns red after a few minutes in the sun it's because it has an intolerance to the chemical filters in the sun cream you are using. Buy a sun cream which doesn't contain any. Also take care with certain medications such as diuretics, antibiotics, anti-inflammatory drugs, antidepressants and certain contraceptive pills. Ask your dermatologist for advice.

KEY FACTS

＊ Take certain precautions: some medicines and chemical filters are allergenic.

＊ Avoid wearing perfume when you are exposed to bright sunlight.

＊ Consult a dermatologist if necessary.

52

try homeopathic remedies

Homeopathy is particularly effective in treating skin disorders, as it targets mind and body simultaneously. It is particularly good for urticaria (hives) and mycosis.

Treat urticaria

Urticaria (hives) are itchy weals or swelling in the skin due to leaky blood vessels. They can have external causes (such as strawberry allergy, sun exposure) or internal (emotional) ones. It takes the form of extremely itchy spots which turn blotchy after a few days then disappear quickly. Homeopathy offers various remedies for urticaria, the most popular of which are listed below:

For each remedy take 3 granules, 4 times per day:
• Itching that worsens on contact with water: *Urtica urens* 9 C.

Red swollen blotches which get better
n cold weather: *Apis* 9 C.

Urticaria arising as a result of exces-
ive eating: *Antimonium crudum* 9 C.

Itching that is alleviated by contact
vith warm water: *Arsenicum album* 9 C.

Combat mycosis

Our skin is host to innumerable bacte-
ia, some of which are essential to our
ealth and well-being. Others, however,
ecome a nuisance when they prolifer-
te. This is the case with the fungus
known as mycosis, which exists in various forms, each of which has a specific
treatment. Here are two of the most
widely used:

• **Dermatophytes:** usually picked up
in the swimming pool or at the sports
hall, and most often found betwen the
toes. Try *Mercurius solubilis* 5 C

• **Candida (oral):** found in the corners
of the lips, often following a course of
antibiotics. Take *Condurango* 4 C.

If this fails there are antibiotic creams
which are also effective in treating these
infections.

KEY FACTS

* Homeopathy is one of the effective ways
to treat urticaria.

* A well-chosen homeopathic remedy can
put an end to even the most stubborn
cases of mycosis.

* For eczema, try consulting a
homeopathic doctor.

53

use Tao for healthy- looking skin

Ancient Chinese doctors felt that a healthy-looking skin reflected the harmony of our inner, vital energy. Today traditional eastern techniques are still used to balance Yin and Yang and improve our outer beauty.

The harmony of Yin and Yang

Ancient Chinese doctors regarded the skin as a mirror of the harmony of our vital energy. Like every other living thing they believed that our body is animated by energy that circulates along channels known as meridians. It has two poles - one called Yin (associated with femininity, gentleness, humidity, the moon and passivity) and the other called Yang (associated with virility, strength, warmth, the sun and activity). Like our health, our beauty is the result of a perfect balance between these two poles of energy.

Yin energy is responsible for the hydro lipid film on the epidermis; it is the source of the softness, suppleness and transparency in our skin. Yang on the ther hand is responsible for skin tone and cellular regeneration. A deficiency in Yin energy manifests itself in wrinkles and a loosening in the contours of the face. A lack of Yang energy gives rise to unwanted redness and blotches.

Energy renewal

During the day our vital energy circulates between organs according to a well-established rhythm. Each organ has a very precise role to play in our skin. When energy circulates badly in the lung meridian, the skin becomes pale and the chin or forehead break out in small spots. When the circulation is poor along the kidney meridian, rings and bags appear beneath the eyes. When circulation along the intestinal meridian is sluggish, the skin becomes red and blotchy with rosacea.

According to eastern traditions, the remedy for such conditions lies in energetic massages or in acupuncture. Plants can also be used in treatments, and changes in diet are also advised, again based on the flow of energy.

● ● ● DID YOU KNOW?

Try Chinese energetic massage known as 'do-in' to revive your skin. Use the fingertips to massage your face.

Start with four points aligned with your eyebrows.

Then work from the centre of your forehead along your nose.

Apply gentle pressure three times on each eye to brighten your eyes.

Massage around your lower lip, starting at the corners.

Repeat each of the above steps five times before moving to the next step.

KEY FACTS

* In Chinese medicine, the skin's beauty is a reflection of the balance of our vital energy.

* Yin and Yang must be in harmony to achieve healthy skin.

54 cure with trace elements

Trace elements really can cure certain problem skin conditions: these substances play a major role in maintaining the health of our skin.

Uses of trace elements The trace elements, which are commonly used by the big cosmetic companies in treatment creams, can also be consumed in their natural forms. They act as enzymes in the millions of biochemical reactions indispensible to cell life. Without them the body and the skin inevitably suffer.

Trace elements à la carte:
• **Copper** helps in the elimination of the free radicals responsible for ageing.
• **Sulphur** is excellent for psoriasis.
• **Manganese** helps combat urticaria and various skin allergies.
• **Lithium** regulates the nervous system and improves skin conditions associated with anxiety and stress.
• **Silicon** is naturally present in the structure of collagen and elastin. It is good for getting rid of warts.

K E Y   F A C T S

* Trace elements are essential to cell life.

* Each one has its own particular properties.

* They are available from pharmacies.

55 discover the beauty of burdock

Herbal therapy was without doubt the first medicine used by man. Scientists are well aware of its efficacy. From the dermatological point of view the one herb which has universal appeal is burdock: whether you have acne or eczema or any other skin complaint, it will be sure to alleviate your symptoms.

An earthly treasure This plant has been known for centuries as one of the treasures of the earth. It owes its popular name 'the ringworm herb' to its traditional use in treating skin troubles.

A natural antibiotic Thanks to its purgative properties, burdock is effective in treating eczema, acne, impetigo and boils, as well as other skin complaints. It is also a natural antibiotic. It can be used as a herbal tea (50g to a litre/2oz to 1 3/4 pints of boiling water; leave to infuse for 10 minutes and drink 3 times a day), or in capsule form (3 a day). It can also be made into a decoction (25g to a litre/1oz to 1 3/4 pints of water, boil for 3 minutes and leave to stand for 10 minutes) which can be used as a lotion on spots and skin lesions.

● ● ● DID YOU KNOW?

> A burdock decoction is also good for hair loss.
> To make a hair tonic, take 200g (7oz) of burdock root and steep in 200ml (6 1/2 fl oz) of wine vinegar for at least 10 days.

KEY FACTS

* Plants are very effective natural medicines.

* Burdock is the king among treatments for skin disorders.

* It has purging and antibiotic properties.

56

beautiful skin and the menopause

The menopause is not an illness. Yet this stage in every woman's life is not without its little miseries, particularly in terms of the skin. To give back to 50-year-old skin the beauty of a flower, natural methods have yet to be beaten.

Effective prevention

From the menopause onwards, wrinkle and drying up of the mucous membranes are what worry a woman most. The production of collagen and the hydration of the skin drop radically when the body ceases to produce oestrogens, so we need to replace them. Of the trace elements, selenium and itamin E are prescribed as a preventative treatment. In addition you can ydrate the skin and the mucous membranes with body oil: shea tree, Chilean husk rose, macadamia, wheatgerm and loe gel are the ideal mixture which any ood pharmacist should be able to make p for you.

soflavones and linolenic acid

o ensure you have a relatively easy menopause it may be necessary to mody your diet: make sure you get enough oflavones and linolenic acid.

Isoflavones are remarkable plant oxidants which do all they can to hold back the years. They are notably found in soya. For combating dryness, try increasing your consumption of oils containing linolenic acid (soya, walnut and olive) and take a course of fish liver oil capsules at regular intervals. Dryness of the vagina responds well to a vaginal oestrogen cream.

KEY FACTS

* Be prepared for wrinkles and dryness of the mucous membranes.

* Increase your intake of oil and soya at mealtimes.

* Use a massage cream with extract of yam.

57 avoid diets

To have beautiful skin you must make sure your diet is rich in certain foods. The problem with this is that the nutrition required by the skin is often at odds with that of the body seeking to be slimmer.

> You don't stop getting vitamins an
minerals when you are following
diet, but there is a strong chance tha
the reduction in your calorific intak
lowers the quality of the micronutr
ents your body absorbs during a da

Dairy products

We know about the benefits to the skin of the bifidus group of bacteria. These aid the digestion so eliminating spots, and they encourage the absorption of the B group vitamins which are vital for a healthy complexion. If you have given up cheese, cream cheese and yoghurts then you must be sure to replace them with food supplements rich in bifidia bacteria.

Cutting out fat

Perhaps you are cutting out fat from your diet in order to lose weight? This makes sense as far as your figure goes but not unfortunately your skin. Fats are absolutely essential components of the cell membranes and if they are deficient the cells harden, the skin dries out and wrinkles appear. In this case the best thing to do is increase your consumption of vegetable oils. A spoonful of olive, corn or groundnut oil in your salad is enough to help restore the cutaneous barrier. Eating oily fish is also important for the fatty acids they contain. If you are following a very strict diet make sure, nonetheless, that you take enough supplements containing oils: fish, borage, evening primrose oil for example. These are low in calories but excellent for the skin.

KEY FACTS

* If you don't eat dairy products take food supplements containing bifidus bacteria.

* If your diet prohibits the consumption of fat, take oil capsules (evening primrose oil, borage or fish).

* If you are following are low-calorie diet make sure you top up with a course of vitamins and minerals.

> When you're on a diet you tend to feel tired quickly, and this has a definite, negative effect on the appearance of the skin. If this is the case, take a course of vitamins and minerals choosing those of natural origin if possible.

In every culture plants are used to enhance beauty. Women from all over the world have long known their benefits. Why not then steep yourself in the immense reservoir of exotic plants?

58

enhance beauty with exotic plants

Aloe: a panacea from the desert

The women of ancient Egypt used aloe daily for their complexions. Hydrating, calming, repairing, aloe vera belongs to the group of 'succulent' oily plants which grow in the desserts of Texas and Mexico. An excellent cell regenerator, it minimizes the loss of water from the epidermis, increases the production of collagen and elastin and speeds up the healing process in damaged skin.

● ● ● D I D   Y O U   K N O W ?

> Eastern women use green tea to enliven tired skin. Do as the Japanese do, and massage your face with green tea leaves crushed in warm water.

> Green tea can help with rosacea as a result of its rich mineral-salt and trace-element content.